KT-498-695

Birth and Parenting Skills

New Directions in Antenatal Education

Mary L. Nolan PhD MA BA(Hons) RGN

Senior Tutor, The National Childbirth Trust, London, UK

Julie Foster RGN DIPHE Nursing RM BSc Midwifery (Hons)

Midwife, Parent Education Co-Ordinator, Birmingham Women's Health Care NHS Trust, UK

Foreword by

Nola Ishmael OBE

Independent Health Advisor/Nurse Leader,

Formerly, Nursing Officer - Department of Health, UK

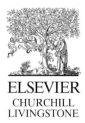

ELSEVIER
CHURCHILL
LIVINGSTONE

EDINBURGH LONDON NEW YORK OXFORD PHILADELPHIA ST LOUIS SYDNEY TORONTO 2005

ELSEVIER
CHURCHILL
LIVINGSTONE

© 2005, Elsevier Limited. All rights reserved.

No part of this publication may be reproduced, stored in a retrieval system, or
transmitted in any form or by any means, electronic, mechanical, photocopying,
recording or otherwise, without either the prior permission of the publishers or a
licence permitting restricted copying in the United Kingdom issued by the
Copyright Licensing Agency, 90 Tottenham Court Road, London W1T 4LP.
Permissions may be sought directly from Elsevier's Health Sciences Rights
Department in Philadelphia, USA: phone: (+1) 215 238 7869, fax: (+1) 215 238 2239,
e-mail: healthpermissions@elsevier.com. You may also complete your request online via the Elsevier homepage (http://www.elsevier.com), by selecting
'Customer Support' and then 'Obtaining Permissions'.

First published 2005

ISBN 0 443 074747

British Library Cataloguing in Publication Data
A catalogue record for this book is available from the British Library

Library of Congress Cataloging in Publication Data
A catalog record for this book is available from the Library of Congress

Note
Knowledge and best practice in this field are constantly changing. As new research
and experience broaden our knowledge, changes in practice, treatment and drug
therapy may become necessary or appropriate. Readers are advised to check the
most current information provided (i) on procedures featured or (ii) by the
manufacturer of each product to be administered, to verify the recommended dose
or formula, the method and duration of administration, and contraindictions. It is
the responsibility of the practitioner, relying on their own experience and
knowledge of the patient, to make diagnoses, to determine dosages and the best
treatment for each individual patient, and to take all appropriate safety
precautions. To the fullest extent of the law, neither the publisher nor the editors
assumes any liability for any injury and/or damage.

The Publisher

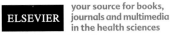
your source for books,
journals and multimedia
in the health sciences

www.elsevierhealth.com

The
publisher's
policy is to use
**paper manufactured
from sustainable forest**

Printed in China

Contents

Contributors

Tom Beardshaw BSc (Econ)(LSE) MTh(Cardiff)
Fathers Direct, Cardiff, UK

Adrienne Burgess BA (Hons)
Policy and Research, Fathers Direct, Byron Bay, Australia

Sheena Byrom RN RM MA
Consultant Midwife Public Health, Queen's Park Hospital, Blackburn, UK

Lorna Davies RN RM PGCEA BSc (Hons) MA
Senior Lecturer in Midwifery, Anglia Polytechnic University, UK

Julie Foster RGN DIPHE Nursing RM BSc Midwifery (Hons)
Midwife, Parent Education Coordinator, Birmingham Women's Health Care NHS Trust, UK

Clare Harding MA (Cantab) MEd DipHE (Antenatal Teaching)
Senior Tutor, The National Childbirth Trust, UK

Willie Henderson MA (Glas) MA (Sussex) DPhil (Sussex)
Director: Centre for Lifelong Learning, University of Birmingham, UK

Mary Nolan PhD MA BA (Hons) RGN
Senior Tutor, The National Childbirth Trust, UK

Alexandra Smith PGCE in Adult Education
Senior Tutor, The National Childbirth Trust, UK

Sara Wickham RM MA BA (Hons) PGCE(A)
Senior Lecturer in Midwifery, Anglia Polytechnic University, UK

Foreword

From time to time, you may see press reports about a 'father of the year' award or an account of a woman described as an 'exceptional mother of the decade'. We read reports in the newspapers that testify to the capability and success of individuals in the parenting role. No single event has made these people successful; instead you read a chronology of events with each one building up the picture of a good parent. On the other hand, it seems that a single incident is sufficient to determine the failure of a parent when that incident is negative.

This begs the question of what constitutes 'best parenting'? What are the set criteria? What portfolio of skills is needed to achieve excellence in parenting? Clearly these questions will generate different answers in different cultures and groups in society. It is important that there are places where the topic can be explored: in parent groups and antenatal classes, in professional settings and forums, in the media via newspapers, magazines and broadcast programmes and in homes between those newly achieving parenthood or those contemplating it.

In fact, parenting is a perennial topic and a perpetual learning curve. It is a lifelong learning activity for which no formal qualifications are demanded. Graduating from the 'school of parenting' is a continuum rather than an achievement and there is never a graduating ceremony. Nonetheless, there are key stages on this lifelong journey and the antenatal period is an important one. In *Birth and Parenting Skills:*

New Directions in Antenatal Education, Mary Nolan, Julie Foster and colleagues explore the vital role of antenatal education in helping prepare women and men for parenthood. The pertinent case is made for 'an empowering philosophy of education for birth and early parenting to underpin a vigorous antenatal programme centred on the needs of families as defined by the families themselves.'

Each chapter explores key points for professionals aiming to provide sound antenatal education. Above all, this excellent book addresses areas that midwives, health visitors, antenatal teachers, childbirth and parenting educators will need to reassess in order to achieve that effectiveness which will be the hallmark of care in 21st century health services. This is a world where parents have many choices, access to a varied menu of electronic information and where the concepts of the *professional* and the *expert* are no longer interchangeable and neither is seen as the fount of all knowledge.

The messages in *Birth and Parenting Skills: New Directions in Antenatal Education* are clear and direct. The challenge is now to rethink the traditional, reform the approaches and redirect the focus in education and learning. I am delighted to be associated with this work and wholeheartedly commend it to you.

Nola Ishmael OBE
Independent Health Advisor / Nurse Leader
Formerly, Nursing Officer – Department of
Health, UK, 2005

Preface

It is very strange that at a time when government is seeking to involve users of services ever more closely in their own care, at a time when education for health and for responsible use of health services is seen as a priority, antenatal education for birth and parenting is being downgraded or abandoned by an increasing number of Trusts. For years, we have been told by midwives, health visitors, educationalists and researchers that pregnancy is a 'teachable moment', a rare, perhaps unique opportunity to engage adults in evaluating their lifestyles and reflecting on their life choices. For a brief period, women and men open themselves to learning when many had battened down the educational hatches after leaving school or completing university, with the feeling that that part of their lives was now complete. Why is it, then, that this precious moment for education, for nurturing parenting and decision-making skills, for strengthening the knowledge base on which people make choices about their own health and that of their families, for enhancing the relationships between parents and their children, why is it that this moment is being overlooked?

Could it be that the commitment to an informed, critical mass of health-care consumers, to an informed electorate, is mere rhetoric? That the development of such a critical mass threatens the power base, the cosy territorialism of all sorts of professionals? Could it be that a critical mass of women and men accessing the maternity care services would demand a very different type of service from the one which is currently available to them? Recent video analysis[1] of interactions in the delivery room suggests that a patriarchal system of care in which the woman and her family are humiliated, ignored and disempowered is still, even in the 21st century, very much alive and well within our hospitals.

It has often been remarked that while training and education are on offer in every work place, there is still virtually no training or education for the most important and influential job that many of us will ever undertake, that of bringing up our children. The antenatal period is clearly the ideal time for making a vigorous start to the education of the nation's parents, so why is it that there is no provision, or that the provision is poor? Is it because its value is not recognised, or because neither the acute nor the community Trusts wish to pay for it? Is it because the only people seen as able to deliver it are midwives and health visitors and these personnel are in very short supply indeed?

As editors of a book on antenatal education, we feel rather like prophets crying from a particularly barren wilderness. Yet we continue to ask the questions. Why is education for birth and parenting important? If it is important, as we believe it is, is it being done well? If it is being done badly, why is this? How could it be improved? Who could improve it? What kind of commitment is needed from commissioners of services, managers and practitioners in order to maximise its potential? Can we afford not to afford antenatal education?

There are some answers in this book. The authors are health professionals, educationalists, childbirth educators and representatives of consumer organisations. They are people who know the value of education in pregnancy because they have been involved in delivering it or preparing others to deliver it for many years; because they are, for the most part, parents and have been consumers of services themselves. They speak with an authoritative voice.

If we are determined to walk the talk, to do something concrete to educate a critical mass of health-care consumers and, ultimately, of voters, then we could do worse than to focus on the antenatal period. In our schools, education for citizenship is now firmly established in the personal, social and health education curriculum because we need good citizens who will take responsibility for nurturing the next generation of good citizens. It surely makes sense to continue education for citizenship after school days are over by providing a birth and parenting curriculum during the special nine months of pregnancy, and, indeed, continuing into the early years of parenting.

This book tackles both the *Why?* of antenatal education and the *How?* It describes innovative and effective practice in different parts of the country, and with different groups of parents. It is, above all, enthusiastic and the editors hope that this enthusiasm will sustain the many people whose contributions to antenatal education are so often dismissed as unimportant in the wider maternity and education services.

Mary Nolan and Julie Foster, 2005

Reference

1. Harris M, Greene K R 2002 How good communication and support – or their absence – affect labour outcomes. The Rising Caesarean Rate 2002: From Audit to Action. Royal College of Physicians, London, p15-18

Acknowledgements

The people to whom we, as editors, writers and, above all, as parent education practitioners, are most indebted in the production of this book are the midwives and childbirth educators who, over many years, have shared their experiences of leading classes and discussion groups with us, and the mothers and fathers who have given us forthright, honest feedback about the classes they have attended! In addition to this considerable body of people are some specific individuals who have not been named in the book, but who deserve to be named here, with gratitude and admiration. The four sections in Chapter 7 attributed to the editors are based on long conversations with people who have shown that parent education is relevant not only to a stereotypical group of educated, middle class mothers, but can also respond to the needs of so-called 'hard-to-reach' groups and make a real difference to their experience of birth and early parenting. Angela McBennett set up, ran, and evaluated the Bellevue Project in Birmingham. Sarah-Jane Watkinson spoke to us at length about her work as Programme Manager with SAMPAD and the antenatal sessions that she helped organise for pregnant women from a south Asian background. The Albany Midwifery Practice's parent education programme was described to us by Pauline Armstrong, the Practice Manager, who also supplied us with a wonderful video of a class in action. And Lizzie Smith spent several hours on the phone, and a few more communicating by email, to tell us about her very successful 4U classes for young mums in the West Midlands. As one of the aims of this book is to advance good practice in parent education, the contributions of these four women, and of Clare Harding, Sheena Byrom and Alexandra Smith who wrote their own sections for Chapter 7, are at the very heart of our enterprise.

Finally, we would like to mention especially Hilary Schmidt-Hansen who spearheaded the South Warwickshire campaign to reinstate parent education classes after they were withdrawn from the local hospital and community, and whose inspiration was very much to the fore in the writing of this book.

Chapter 1

Childbirth and Parenting Education:

what the research says and why we might ignore it

Mary Nolan

The book starts by reviewing the literature around antenatal education for birth and parenting. The author finds that the quality of the research is seriously flawed and argues that we can draw very few conclusions from it about the value of antenatal education in helping women and their partners cope with the challenges of labour and birth, and the transition to parenthood. Instead, she suggests that we look at developing an empowering philosophy of education for birth and early parenting to underpin a vigorous antenatal education programme which is centred on the needs of families as defined by themselves.

(Editors' note)

Education is generally considered to be 'a good thing', so are we to presume that, by implication, education for childbirth and parenting must also be a good thing? Have we any proof that it is? Are we absolutely sure that it is worth giving our time and commitment to it?

What are we trying to achieve through education for birth and parenting? Unless we have a very clear idea about how we would answer this question, we really shouldn't be out there practising. We cannot impose a curriculum on an audience as vulnerable, and as eager to learn as expectant parents if we haven't reflected at some length on what that curriculum should be and why teaching those subject areas and those skills is important.

People come to antenatal classes primarily to find out about labour and giving birth. They also have a parenting agenda which may, or generally may not, be met. However, taking it as a given that birth is their main concern, the first question childbirth educators have to answer is what their aim is in preparing parents for birth. Is it best to prepare them for consultant unit birth, or are we going to try and prepare them for normal birth (presuming that those two things are generally not synonymous)? If the thrust of the curriculum is going to be towards helping parents achieve a normal birth, are we sure that we know what that is? Has the hospital in which we work a definition of normal birth? I know of units which lay claim to operate a midwifery model of birth where clients are accepted for induction, epidurals are available 24/7 and ventouse deliveries are carried out. If our definition of *normal* birth includes all these interventions, how does our curriculum cater for those parents who would like a birth without any medication or interventions?

If we consider normal birth to be:

- A birth that starts spontaneously
- A birth in which the mother is upright, mobile and chooses her own positions
- A birth in which the interplay of prostaglandins, oxytocin, adrenalin and endorphins is allowed to happen freely
- A birth in which the mother is supported throughout by the physical and emotional care of her chosen birth companions
- A birth in which the mother pushes her baby out into the world through her own, unaided efforts
- A birth after which the mother and baby are alert and ready to engage in instinctive bonding and attachment behaviours

and if we believe that the majority of women are physically able to achieve such a birth, we will lead classes which are very different from those provided by an educator whose concept of normality includes a range of medical procedures. We must define what it is we are trying to achieve in order to be able to evaluate whether we have achieved it and plan for how we can do better.

It is rare for researchers studying childbirth and parenting education to ask educators for what kind of birth they are preparing women and their companions. It is equally rare for researchers to ask educators what their underpinning philosophy of adult education is, to what educational principles they adhere, what criteria they use to evaluate their classes – indeed, whether they have ever thought at all about why they are doing what they are doing.

The influence of teachers is legendary. It is therefore only ethical for teachers to have a clear idea of the direction in which that influence will be working. How childbirth educators feel about birth and how they define normal birth will influence the kind of language they use, the teaching strategies they employ and the relationship they establish with the parents who attend classes. If educators don't believe normal birth is particularly desirable or achievable within an acute hospital environment, the words they use to describe birth and medical procedures, and the ways in which they portray the role of labouring women and their birth companions will be different from those of

Table 1.1 Relationship between the educator's philosophy, the curriculum and teaching approaches

Centre of classes	Curriculum	Teaching approaches
Birth as it is at this hospital (induction rate: 26%; augmentation rate: 20%; epidural rate: 68%; assisted delivery rate: 20%; caesarean section rate: 24%)	Induction: why and how; failure to progress; EFM - intermittent and continuous; epidural analgesia - procedure, benefits (? and hazards); assisted delivery - why and how, benefits (? and hazards); caesarean section - why and how, benefits (? and hazards)	Lectures to give information; minimal opportunity for discussion; no practice of self-help skills for labour; birth companion peripheral to classes; classes delivered to large groups
Normal birth (starts spontaneously; not augmented; without pethidine or epidural; spontaneous delivery)	How the baby moves through the pelvis; effect of pregnancy hormones on pelvic elasticity; effect of upright positions and mobility on progress of labour; role of birth companion; eating and drinking in labour; late first stage – the physical and emotional experience; positions for effective pushing; typical behaviour of the newborn baby	Demonstrations by educator; multiple opportunities for parents to practise self-help skills; frequent discussion of emotions; birth companion central to classes; classes delivered to small groups

colleagues who do think most women are able to achieve a normal birth. Their educational aims will be different if they find the active management of labour a sensible and compassionate approach to birth and therefore ally themselves with the many doctors who consider labour a medical crisis or inconvenience which they must – *in their role as experts … cure as soon as possible* (Budin, 2001:39).

The kind of education which the educator provides will reflect her concept of women's powerfulness or powerlessness in childbirth. Childbirth educators must make a decision about whether they place at the centre of their classes birth as it is normally experienced in their unit, or normal birth. The effect on the curriculum and teaching approaches will be dramatic (see Table 1.1).

Wherever we are 'coming from' in terms of our philosophy of birth, we cannot be ethical educators if we have not reflected on and to some extent formalised our understanding of the purpose of childbirth education. It may not be necessary to have a written mission statement, or series of principles (although the act of writing ideas down certainly helps to tighten up thinking) but it is essential to be able to give a coherent and thoughtful account of what it is we are doing.

There is much in the literature from the New World (and some from the 'Old') that educators can use to help structure their thinking and empower them in their work. In the States, teachers trained in the Lamaze method deliver a significant proportion of childbirth education. These teachers work within the health-care system as well as independently of it. The Lamaze organisation is clear about its philosophy of birth:

- Birth is normal, natural and healthy
- The experience of birth profoundly affects women and their families
- Women's inner wisdom guides them through birth
- Women's confidence and ability to give birth is either enhanced or diminished by the care provider and place of birth
- Women have the right to give birth free from routine medical interventions
- Birth can take place in birth centers and homes
- Childbirth education empowers women to make informed choices in health care, to assume responsibility for their health, and to trust their inner wisdom.

(http://www.lamaze.org/2000/about_lamaze.html)

> *Ultimately the goal of Lamaze classes is that every woman gives birth confidently, free to find comfort in a wide variety of ways, and supported by family and health care professionals who trust that she has within her the ability to give birth.*
>
> *(Lamaze International, 2002)*

The Australian literature discusses a 'family-centred' philosophy of childbirth education (Rolls & Cutts, 2001:54), and in the States, a Family-Centered Perinatal Education Program (Haskins Westmoreland & Zwelling, 2000) is considered to:

- Prepare families for active participation throughout the evolving process of preconception, pregnancy, childbirth and parenting
- Assist the family in making informed choices for their care during pregnancy, labor and birth, and for postpartum/newborn care
- Actively involve the father and/or other supportive person(s) in the educational process
- Address the long-term emotional significance of the childbearing experience
- Reflect the cultural needs of the participants
- Facilitate the group process, with an ideal size of 6–10 couples and a maximum of 12 couples
- Include discussion of consumer rights and responsibilities for making informed choice based on knowledge of alternatives
- Actively seek family input and evaluation of class content and process in order to improve classes.

From Germany comes a concept of the content and nature of childbirth education which demands humility, self-awareness, sensitivity and intelligence on the part of the educator:

Gesellschaft fur Geburtsvorbereitung

The course curriculum

- includes emotional, cognitive/informative and social aspects of birth, and their integral connection within group processes
- relates the physical aspects of birth to the possibility of a deeper experiencing of one's own body, with the purpose of building trust in one's own capabilities and strength
- supports individual coping strategies for facing the undefined birth experience.

Essential features of the course are:

- the explicit, continuous inclusion of the partner within the framework of couple courses
- closed groups with permanent primary instructors. *Only so can a trusting, open atmosphere arise in which the supportive, sharing and creative potential of the group can be awakened.* (Müller-Staffelstein, 1996:74)

Childbirth educators in the UK have been slow to formulate and broadcast what it is they have to offer to childbearing families which is not provided by other professional groups. Yet as collaborative working comes increasingly under scrutiny, professional groups are being asked to define exactly what it is they are contributing to the team effort. In a climate of cost-cutting and demands for proofs of effectiveness, the starting point for preservation of one's profession must be the ability to state clearly what is unique about its approach to care and what are the particular skills of its members.

A review of the literature on the effectiveness of childbirth education reveals that, for the most part, the aims of the childbirth educators or their programmes were never made clear to the researchers (and perhaps weren't clear to the educators themselves). The outcomes measured have generally been the hard outcomes (number of hours in labour; uptake of epidural anaesthesia; operative delivery rate; breastfeeding success) which researchers have assumed – without asking either the educators or the parents attending the classes – are appropriate to childbirth education. Yet the learning that can be measured using a quantitative analysis is very limited indeed.

The value of the research is further diminished by its total disregard of the circumstances under which parents attempt to implement the learning they have achieved. Lamaze classes, and those provided in the UK by educators from the National Childbirth Trust, emphasise the importance of continuous emotional and physical support in labour, something that most busy (or even averagely busy) maternity units cannot provide. Even if there were more staff on duty, it is by no means certain that they have the skills to provide this kind of support, or even

Table 1.2 Women's expectations and experiences of midwives (Spiby et al, 1999)

	What women wanted (n=121)	Women's perceptions of midwife's involvement in labour	
To prompt	115 (95%)	30 (25%)	(1)
		27 (35%)	(2)
To encourage	117 (97%)	50 (41%)	(1)
		77 (64%)	(2)
To demonstrate	93 (77%)	18 (15%)	(1)
		28 (23%)	(2)

(1) = first midwife involved in care in labour
(2) = second midwife involved in care in labour

that they want to. Working with a group of first year midwifery students recently, we engaged in a discussion on the nature and extent of care that midwives offer to childbearing women. One student said she thought it was unreasonable and unrealistic to expect midwives to provide care in any domain other than the physical. Many students were in agreement with her. If the ethos of midwifery care is so restricted, birth environments will inevitably frustrate childbirth educators *in their efforts to help women develop and maintain confidence in their ability to give birth* (Lamaze International, 2002:2). Education for normal birth will fail if the woman is not supported *by health care professionals who trust that she has within her the ability to give birth* (p 3) As Madeleine Shearer (1990) aptly commented – delivery suite staff have an almost limitless capacity to make childbirth education seem relevant and useful, or to make it seem out-of-touch and ridiculous.

Recent research by Spiby and colleagues (1999) into whether antenatal education translates into practice reports that when women class attenders looked ahead to their labours, they stated that they hoped their midwives would 'prompt' them in the use of coping strategies, 'encourage' them and 'demonstrate' to them. Table 1.2 shows what really happened.

Spiby speculates as to why midwives did not support the class attenders in implementing the self-help skills they had practised antenatally. She wonders whether there was a lack of confidence on the midwives' part in women's ability to cope with labour. She suggests that midwives may be hesitant about intruding on a woman and her birth companion when all appears to be going well, but acknowledges that unobtrusive support at least should be provided. Interestingly, her study concludes that there is a need for a revised programme of antenatal education rather than a revised approach to care in the delivery room!

Where childbirth educators are unsure of what they are teaching (normal birth/hospital birth) and why they are teaching it (empowerment/conformity), and when the environment of birth fails to support the skills women and their companions have acquired in antenatal classes, much research into the outcomes of childbirth education can be seen to have been pointless.

For the most part, studies carried out prior to Spiby's work considered the effect of antenatal classes primarily in terms of the number of interventions in labour that women who have attended classes undergo, or their uptake of pharmacological forms of pain relief. Green et al's overview (1988) of studies from the 1970s and early 1980s, while being generally critical of the methodologies employed and aware of the very different teaching approaches deployed in the classes attended by subjects, concludes:

> One consistent finding is that women trained in childbirth education use less analgesia and anaesthesia than untrained women. (1:4)

The majority of later studies have, for reasons that will be apparent from what has already been said in this chapter, found *no* differences between groups of class attenders and control groups of non-attenders. In 1983, Gunn et al studied nearly 200 mothers in Auckland, half of whom attended classes and half of whom did not. The researchers found no significant difference between the groups in terms of their use of drugs for pain relief in labour, and an equal number in both groups were reported as being disappointed with their birth experience. Copstick et al (1985) looked at the efficacy of breathing and postural techniques taught at antenatal classes and found that the overwhelming majority of mothers did not make use of them during labour. An American study by Whipple et al (1990) investigated ten women, five of whom had attended Lamaze classes and the other five no classes, and found that the prepared women managed pain more effectively. Their assessment of pain control was made by subjecting the women – during labour – to a finger prick of increasing intensity. The researchers concluded that the effectiveness of childbirth preparation was undeniable in the prepared group! The ethics of this study coupled with its limitations in terms of sample size make its results questionable to say the least.

Hetherington's study (1990) of women attending classes at an inner-city hospital in Baltimore is rare in the annals of research into childbirth preparation because more than half the subjects were black and the majority were poor women without private medical insurance. This study matched women who chose to attend classes with a control group who chose not to on the variables of race, patient status (clinic or private), parity, marital status and age. Far less analgesia was used by the study group who also achieved more spontaneous deliveries (two factors which are, of course, not unrelated). Hetherington considers various factors which might have influenced her results apart from the content and teaching approaches of the classes. She speculates whether self-esteem was an important variable in making some women seek childbirth preparation, and whether it was that self-esteem that subsequently influenced their choice of pain relief in labour (rather than the classes they had attended). She also questions whether there might have been differences between the two groups for which the study could not control, such as whether the women who took classes were inherently more capable of making decisions and relying on their own resources during labour than the control group women.

Redman et al's study (1991) carried out in Australia, found that women greatly enjoyed the classes they attended, but that antenatal education did not impact on their behaviour during labour nor influence the kind of pain relief that they used. The study by Lumley and Brown (1993) replicated the results of their co-patriots, finding that attendance at classes was not associated with differences in birth events or satisfaction among women having their first child.

Sturrock and Johnson's research (1990) concluded that 114 well-educated, high socio-economic status, older women who attended classes at the Hays Army Community Hospital were at a *disadvantage* in terms of their experience of labour when compared with a control group of younger, less socially privileged non-attenders. Thirty-eight per cent of the women who had been to classes had a caesarean section compared with 29% of the control women, while the length of second stage was 1.07 hours in the intervention group and 0.79 hours in the control group. The authors relate outcomes purely to attendance at classes, although with such an astronomically high rate of caesarean section, one is bound to speculate about what was going on in the delivery suite! It might also be asked whether the high socio-economic status of the women class attenders resulted in their having more attention – in the form of intervention – than their less socially exalted sisters. The relationship between wealth and birth by the abdominal route is well documented throughout the world (Wagner, 1994).

Qureshi et al's paper appeared in 1996. This study investigated 155 class attenders and 88 non-attenders and reported that although 145 women found the classes useful or very useful, there were no differences between the groups in terms of the amount or type of analgesia the women used during labour. The researchers did not ask the women why they had found the classes useful, or engage in any speculation on such an interesting anomaly. Clearly, their outcome measures were not the only ones of interest to the women who, it would appear, gained something from the classes other than what could be measured quantitatively.

This paper is symptomatic of the almost universal assumption made by researchers that women's agenda in attending classes is solely to learn about pain relief in labour and medical interventions. Research into what women and their partners and families want from antenatal education is limited and it is by no means clear that the little we do know about their preferred agenda currently informs childbirth preparation programmes. Studies from the early 90s reveal that women are interested in issues extending well beyond labour and pain relief. Redman et al (1991) noted that class attenders valued the information they gained about sources of support for after the birth. Hillan (1992) found that women wanted much more information in classes on deviations from the normal course of labour, on perineal pain and on how to recognise and manage postnatal depression. Women's need for more and better education in preparation for parenting is made clear by several studies (Gould, 1986; Hillan, 1992; O'Meara, 1993; Nolan, 1997). The same theme has reappeared in the more recent literature with Schneider (2001) finding that women were as interested in baby care, coping with a new infant at home and breastfeeding as they were in labour and pain relief, yet the postnatal agenda was inadequately covered:

> All the women said the information on labour, birth and pain relief was relevant and helpful. Most were disappointed that they received so little information on baby care and coping with an infant in the early days ... They wanted more information about infant care and handling; communication; patterns of behaviour (e.g. crying, feeding, sleeping); about how they may feel physically and emotionally in the early days at home (p16,18).

These women's agenda was also very much a social one, both in the sense of wanting to meet people in a similar situation and being able to share time with their partner (p15). The opportunity for couples attending classes to grow in understanding of each other's ideas and needs has been given little, if any, attention in the literature.

There is some guidance as to what men want from antenatal classes. Nolan's study (1994) of men attending classes provided by the National Childbirth Trust found that they wanted information about labour and especially about how they could help their partners; they also wanted to know what they could do to help after the birth and how they could be involved in caring for their baby. In defining exactly what aspects of the postnatal period most occupy men, Matthey et al's study (2002) is very helpful. Men are interested in:

- the responsibility of becoming a parent
- whether they or their partners will struggle to cope with being a parent
- whether they and their partners will be good enough parents
- whether their partners might get lonely or bored at home
- the effect of parenthood on their work

- feeding and changing the baby; baby's sleep patterns
- the cost of having a baby.

Some men are concerned about how the arrival of the baby will affect their relationship with their own parents. Haskins Westmoreland and Zwelling (2000) recommend *an in-depth community needs assessment … to identify the classes desired by families* (p33). Teaching to the kind of 'standardized programme' which Spiby et al (1999) describe in their research is never likely to satisfy parents. It is always unwise for educators to presume that they know what parents want, and if they have been leading classes for many years, it is even more unwise for them to make this assumption. Camiletti's and Alder's study (1999) of an agenda for early pregnancy classes found a considerable gap between the topics that women stated they were most interested in and those cited by midwives. The women were very concerned about environmental health issues:

- Safety of caffeine and herbal teas
- Folic acid/iron/calcium/vitamin supplements
- Computer monitors/video display terminals
- Saunas/hot tubs
- Paint fumes
- Insecticides
- Radiation/electro-magnetic fields.

These topics ranked in the top 20 of the 45 topics the women were asked to list in order of preference for an early pregnancy class. They were very rarely included in the traditional prenatal curriculum in Ontario where the study was carried out.

Why it is that childbirth and parent educators continue to assert that their clients are not interested in anything beyond labour and birth is difficult to understand given the weight of research showing that expectant parents are *extremely* interested in postnatal issues. There may be a number of reasons why educators shy away from the parenting component of the antenatal course, and cite parental indifference as a reason for lack of inclusion of key postnatal topics. The process of labour is easily described; much of the information that parents need is factual – the signs of early labour; what happens in the first/second/third stages; how the baby's heartbeat is monitored; how labour is induced and augmented; what is involved in a forceps, ventouse or caesarean delivery. Midwives and health visitors are confident that they have this kind of information at their fingertips. The issues around parenting are much more to do with how individuals adapt to the unpredictability of baby routines; how relationships change when a baby comes into the family; how work and family life can be reconciled; how women adjust to an altered body image and role, and how their partners adjust. These are issues to which there is no right or wrong answer; they demand teaching and learning in the affective rather than the cognitive domain.

They are consequently topics that are much more difficult to teach, demand much greater insight and self-awareness on the part of the educator, and are energy-consuming. The educator is not 'the expert' because there is no factual base to parenting, but only the individual's and the couple's take on it. All the educator can do is help each person develop his or her understanding of the transition to parenthood within the context of his or her own life. It may be that educators are much less comfortable with this role than with telling parents what happens in labour.

The literature rarely makes clear whether childbirth preparation and parent education classes taking place in the antenatal period are founded on a model of adult education. Adults will not learn if they are not treated as adults – with acknowledgment of the mass of experience they already have of themselves, of life and of facing and overcoming challenges – and respected for their autonomous status as people who can make their own decisions:

> In fact, the psychological definition of adult is 'one who has arrived at a self-concept of being responsible for one's own life, of being self-directing'. When we have arrived at that point, we develop a deep psychological need to be perceived by others, and treated by others, as capable of taking responsibility for ourselves. (Knowles, 1984:9)

Angela Underdown (1998) carried out a courageous and revealing piece of work in which she investigated whether health professionals demonstrate effective group facilitation skills when teaching antenatal classes. Ten classes, each led by a different educator, were observed. The verbal interactions during the classes were sampled and coded, and a questionnaire asking the educators for information about previous experience and training was distributed. Underdown noted that:

- 90% of the classes were directive in approach
- More than 75% of the questions asked by educators were closed, and 78% of the parents' responses were restricted
- Seven of the ten classes showed a high level of teacher input, and a low level of acceptance of parents' ideas, behaviours and feelings
- Eight of the ten classes started late
- Most of the teachers did not know all of the clients by name
- Four of the ten classes were interrupted, inhibiting the creation of a safe group environment
- Videos were used as 'fillers' rather than as pertinent teaching tools.

Underdown is extremely sympathetic towards the health professionals who participated in her study, 80% of whom reported that they had received only four hours instruction, or less, on the theory of group work in their initial training. Yet she concludes that *there were many lost learning opportunities and the educators' directive approach was a barrier in helping to address the real needs of the client* (p67).

It may be that even when health professionals are genuinely skilled as educators of adults, they are not allowed to make education the *'practice of freedom', the means by which men and women deal critically and creatively with reality and discover how to participate in the transformation of their world* (Freire, 1972). Subtle or not so subtle pressure may be exerted on them to educate parents for compliance with hospital protocols and procedures or in accordance with *professional idealist beliefs* (Hancock, 1994). Informed choice may be the rhetoric of managers, but actively discouraged in practice. In the States, the autonomy of educators to practise in accordance with generally accepted principles of adult education is regularly challenged within a health care system that is heavily weighted in favour of the priorities and preferences of doctors:

> *In Ohio, a childbirth education association was kicked out of a hospital because a provider didn't want women to hear that episiotomy is not always necessary ... An educator at another faculty was told, not asked, by an obstetric resident, to teach more about epidurals because he needed practice with his forceps. (Lee, 1999:40)*

The author, a nurse and childbirth educator, was told by her managers that *if anything untoward occurs during the birth, women should feel it was inevitable* (p40) and that she should focus less on emotions and choices, less on risks and more on facts.

If, over the years, educators have, knowingly or otherwise, been educating for compliance, then the results of the research which has assessed whether antenatal classes impact on interventions in labour prove that classes have been *extremely successful* – the research has shown the intervention rate to be no different for class attenders than for non-attenders.

If the hidden agenda is to ensure a high uptake of interventions which are delivered by doctors, with epidurals as the most obvious of these, then a didactic, directive approach to classes will be the most successful. An adult education approach which encourages and assists parents to reflect on their own needs and on how best to fulfil them, which promotes independent thinking and a questioning attitude, will not be welcomed within an ethos of education for dependence. *If the medium is the message* (Simkin & Enkin, 1989) and the message is compliance, the content of antenatal education should ideally not be dictated by parents, and the process should not be learner-centred. A prescriptive format for classes, with unlimited numbers of participants, and no exchange between parents and educators meets the political agenda perfectly:

A 7 week childbirth series was offered, which consisted of a 2 hour class on each of the following topics: (a) childbirth preparation for labor, (b) relaxation techniques and a tour of the maternity care facilities, (c) postpartum and caesarean birth, (d) breastfeeding, (e) vaginal birth after caesarean, (f) siblings and (g) newborn care. The number of participants in these classes was not limited and classes were held in a large auditorium ... Hospital tours had as many as 70 people attending, with one instructor as guide. The class hand-outs were sporadic and of inconsistent quality. (Haskins Westmoreland and Zwelling, 2000)

In 1999, the Royal College of Midwives, recognising that the quality of education for childbirth and parenting in the UK was poor, issued a series of booklets designed to assist midwives in leading antenatal classes. The venture failed because the booklets addressed only the content of classes (and the heavy emphasis on psychoanalytic theory bore little relevance to the needs of parents as they themselves might see them) and not the process. This was a missed opportunity – what was required was a vigorous assessment of why childbirth and parenting education was failing, with an examination of the professional and health care context in which it was being provided. Has the UK ever undertaken the kind of hard-hitting appraisal which was carried out in Australia a few years ago? The New South Wales Standing Committee on Social Issues (1998) criticised childbirth and parent education programmes for their:

- Didactic approach
- Large groups
- Failure to address the learning needs identified by participants
- Lack of involvement of male participants and recognition of their needs
- Failure to prepare women and men for the emotional and psychological aspects of parenthood.

Margaret Mason (1997), writing of the obstacles to woman-centred classes in Dublin, focuses attention on some of the most important issues for providers:

- Lack of integration of childbirth and parent education with other aspects of the maternity services
- Philosophical conflicts – differing models of care and lack of respect for the skills of others hindering an unbiased approach to childbirth education
- Lack of teaching skills, particularly in adult education.

Such clear-sighted understanding of the problems, and the courage to articulate them uncompromisingly, are the first vital steps towards providing education for childbirth and parenting which will truly meet the needs of the large numbers of women and men who seek such education in good faith and deserve a first rate service.

CONCLUSION

The research tells us very little about the effectiveness of antenatal education. It is generally unhelpful, not to say misleading, in terms of defining appropriate outcome measures. For a much better account of what antenatal education might achieve, and may already be achieving when delivered by skilled educators, read Alexandra Smith's chapter (3) later in this book. However, the literature does include some important critical thinking about what is wrong with antenatal education; although it may be that the issues are intractable, they are part of the fabric of the system of health care which we, the people, have created for ourselves and endorsed. Wickham's and Davies' chapter (5) examines whether it is possible to change what is 'rotten in the heart of Denmark'. In the meantime, women and their partners continue to ask for classes and we must use what is already known about an appropriate agenda for antenatal education and the processes which enable adults to learn effectively, to try to provide a service that meets at least some of their needs. Julie Foster's chapter (6) describes an innovative and effective brief educational intervention for childbirth, and Chapter 7 describes other powerful and needs-orientated programmes.

REFERENCES

Budin W C 2001 Birth and death: opportunities for self-transcendence. The Journal of Perinatal Education 10(1):38-42

Camiletti Y A, Alder R 1999 Learning needs as perceived by women less than or equal to 16 weeks pregnant. Canadian Journal of Public Health 90(4):229-232

Copstick S, Hayes R W, Taylor K E et al 1985 A test of a common assumption regarding the use of antenatal training during labour. Journal of Psychosomatic Research 29(2):215-218

Freire P 1972 Pedagogy of the oppressed. Translated by Myra Bergman Ramos. Herder and Herder, New York

Gould D 1986 Locally organised antenatal classes and their effectiveness. Nursing Times 82(45):59-61

Green J M, Coupland V A, Kitzinger J V 1988 Great expectations: a prospective study of women's expectations and experiences of childbirth, Vol. 1. Child Care and Development Group, University of Cambridge

Gunn T R, Fisher A, Lloyd P, O'Donnell S 1983 Antenatal education: does it improve the quality of labour and delivery? New Zealand Medical Journal 96:51-53

Hancock A 1994 How effective is antenatal education? Modern Midwife 4(5):13

Haskins Westmoreland M, Zwelling E 2000 Developing a family-centered, hospital-based perinatal education program. The Journal of Perinatal Education 9(4):28-39

Hetherington S E 1990 A controlled study of the effect of prepared childbirth classes on obstetric outcomes. Birth 17(2):86-90

Hillan E 1992 Issues in the delivery of midwifery care. Journal of Advanced Nursing, 17:274-278

Knowles M 1984 Andragogy in action (Introduction). Jossey-Bass, London

Lamaze International 2002 Position Paper – Lamaze for the 21st century. The Journal of Perinatal Education 11(1): 1-4

Lee N 1999 The missing squatting bar: childbirth education in the '90s. Midwifery Today Summer: 40-43

Lumley J, Brown S 1993 Attenders and nonattenders at childbirth education classes in Australia: How do they and their births differ? Birth 20(3):123-130

Matthey S, Morgan M, Healey L et al 2002 Postpartum issues for expectant mothers and fathers. Journal of Obstetrics, Gynecology and Neonatal Nursing 31(4):428-435

Müller-Staffelstein T 1996 Preparation for childbirth – preparation for life: a challenge for primary prevention. International Journal of Prenatal and Perinatal Psychology and Medicine 8 (suppl):73-79

New South Wales (NSW) Standing Committee on Social Issues 1998 Working for children: communities supporting families. Inquiry into parent education and support programs. New South Wales Government, Sydney, Australia

Nolan M 1994 Caring for fathers in antenatal classes. Modern Midwife 4(2):25-28

Nolan M 1997 Antenatal education: failing to educate for parenthood. British Journal of Midwifery 5(1):21-26

O'Meara C 1993 An evaluation of consumer perspectives of childbirth and parenting education. Midwifery 9(4):210-219

Qureshi N S, Schofield G, Papaioannou S et al 1996 Parentcraft classes: do they affect outcome in childbirth? Journal of Obstetrics and Gynaecology 1(6):358-361

Redman S, Oak S, Booth P et al 1991 Evaluation of an antenatal education programme: characterisitics of attenders, changes in knowledge and satisfaction of participants. Australia and New Zealand Journal of Obstetrics and Gynecology 31(4):310-316

Rolls C, Cutts D 2001 Pregnant-to-parenting education: creating a new approach. Birth Issues 10(2):53-58

Royal College of Midwives 1999 Transition to parenting: an open learning resource for midwives. Royal College of Midwives Trust, London

Schneider Z 2001 Antenatal education classes in Victoria: what the women said. Australian College of Midwives Incorporated 14(3):14-21

Shearer M 1990 Effects of prenatal education depend on the attitudes and practices of obstetric caregivers. Birth 17(2):73-74

Simkin P, Enkin M 1989 Antenatal classes. In: Enkin M, Kierse M, Chalmers I (eds) Effective Care in Pregnancy and Childbirth. Oxford University Press, Oxford, p 318-334

Spiby H, Henderson B, Slade P et al 1999 Strategies for coping with labour: does antenatal education translate into practice? Journal of Advanced Nursing 29(2):388-394

Sturrock W A, Johnson J 1990 The relationship between childbirth education classes and obstetric outcome. Birth 17(2):82-85

Underdown A 1998 Investigating techniques used in parenting classes. Health Visitor 71(2):65-68

Wagner M 1994 Pursuing the birth machine: the search for appropriate birth technology. ACE Graphics, Camperdown, NSW

Whipple B, Josimovich J, Komisaruk B 1990 Sensory thresholds during the antepartum, intrapartum and postpartum periods. International Journal of Nursing Studies 27(3):213-221

Chapter 2

Context and Purpose:
learning styles and principles of adult education

Willie Henderson

A coherent and comprehensive philosophy of antenatal education must encompass an understanding of the nature of adult learning and of the need which adult learners have to be recognised as autonomous individuals, seeking increased adulthood rather than increased dependence. Those running classes or groups for expectant parents should aim to make themselves redundant – to educate parents who can continue the journey of learning on their own. In preparing people for birth and parenting, it is especially important to draw on their previous life experiences, and to link past learning with new, to challenge preconceived ideas and reframe them, and to reflect on what may be the influences on their parenting styles. A pedagogic or 'expert' approach cannot respond to the rich variety of adult learners' experiences and needs and antenatal education is therefore essentially client-led, interactive and dynamic.   *(Editors' note)*

This chapter will start by looking at what principles can be achieved in learning and teaching terms, by reflecting upon 'adult learners in general'. These reflections will give rise to a series of insights that are helpful as a way of engaging in planning a curriculum in a given context. Thinking about adults in general can take us some of the way towards planning an effective curriculum based upon partnership in learning. However, we never teach adults in general, only the particular people who decide to come along to our classes. Getting to know individuals and learning to work with a diversity of experiences and with different learning styles leads to interesting and dynamic educational environments. Understanding the learners' context and purposes is important. Tapping into experience helps us to know the participants. Learning styles, also, are now better formally understood amongst the community of adult educators than they have been in the past. In addition, therefore, this chapter will explore what models of learning those engaged in working with adults, in the context of antenatal education, may draw upon to inform their teaching. What learning styles are there? How are learning styles to be thought about? Are they rigid or developmental? What are the implications for teaching methods? The penultimate section will consider and exemplify the curriculum uses of the Kolb Learning Cycle.

TURNING PARTICIPANTS 'ON' TO LEARNING

Although the word 'adult' is resorted to frequently in conversations about 'adult education' it is, in many respects, an unusual word. In wider society it is often used to refer to explicit knowledge concerning sex and sexuality ('This film contains scenes of an adult nature') or it is used to challenge a put-down ('Do not talk to me like that, I am, after all, an adult') or when being charged for entry to a cinema ('Two adults, one child'). In everyday life many of us are willing to label ourselves in a variety of contexts, professional or otherwise, as having a particular role or function (e.g. midwife, lecturer, parent) but we very rarely label ourselves as 'adults'. Talking about adult education assumes that we *do* and this may not be very helpful, however convenient it is for the educator even if only as shorthand. Participants on educational programmes aimed at 'adults' (in other words people like us) have other images and motivations, other contexts in which they think about themselves (partners; parents; workers; carers; ballroom dancers/singers/hobbyists of a variety of sorts; consumers; friends; members of faith communities; successful/unsuccessful learners – and all the ethical and emotional issues that people bring to such contexts) and their relationship with the programme of study. Their experience, and the contexts in which they come to programmes, are important elements to be tapped into, according to adult education theory, in thinking about many aspects of curriculum development. Teachers do not need to gain access to the whole of this experience but it helps if they can make links between experience and the learning outcomes that are being promoted.

Contexts shape meaning and the meaning of the programme from the individual's point of view is significant. An essential ambiguity to be considered here is that what a tutor teaches is not necessarily what a participant learns. Learning can be considered as a kind of negotiation that goes on within a participant's mind as new knowledge supports or challenges existing knowledge and understanding. Learning can be seen as the resolution of confusion and conflict as existing ideas adjust to accommodate new challenges. Indeed, the notion of adult education itself has been realigned, in recent years, into discussions around themes suggested by 'lifelong learning'. In this model, much of people's everyday behaviour and experiences are understood as learning though the activities take place within life and not school. Thus we learn, largely through experience, to be parents or how to live on our own on the death of a close partner. We engage in a learning process, for example, when trying to decide on where to go on holiday or searching for a new job or buying a new house or a new car. These processes are not normally labelled as 'learning' though this is what they are. Reflecting non-judgementally upon how we go about such learning, compared, say, to a partner or a friend or colleague, can provide us with insight into our own learning style. 'Adult education' often carries with it the image of local authority evening classes (a valuable tradition, in need of some revitalisation), whereas lifelong learning carries within it notions of flexible learning available through formal and non-formal educational contexts, from a variety of institutions and delivered by a variety of methods and taken up in the context of busy lives. So 'lifelong learning' suggests a diversity of provision, of delivery and of contexts.

It is, equally, not always the case that those engaged in teaching adults see themselves as 'adult educators'. The context in which many work and think about their role is likely to be as a professional, first, rather than as an educator. Thus midwives, who teach adults some of the time, may be carrying out a professional role and that role just happens to include some teaching. If the profession tends to be relatively isolated 'on the ground' as it were, then opportunities to discuss their role as educators may be sparse. It would be natural in such contexts for the professional basis for engaging in curriculum design and delivery to be dominant and for insights on the teaching of adults to be based upon experience, or to be at the very least, secondary concerns. Thus, within antenatal education, a starting point is what could be called the 'expert model of delivery', in which the professional is seen to have significant theoretical and practical knowledge that has to be transmitted to the learner. The learner is there to absorb a curriculum that is subject-oriented and expert-led. This model has often been a starting point but has given way to a model of education based on the notion that any programme of study is, or ought to be, a *partnership* between the learner and the educator. Seeing participants as engaging in a programme of personal growth, motivated by questions, aspirations, fears and inadequate experience, and putting these first and subject expertise second in the design of the curriculum is essentially a student-centred approach. Teaching and curriculum design skills required for successful application of the partnership model or for the student-centred model tend to be different from those required in the expert-led model and part of the purpose of this chapter will be to review the skills required.

Broadly speaking, the expert-led model requires expert subject knowledge and suggests a limited role for the exchange of experience and points of view, i.e. for the construction of knowledge and understanding through discussion and exchange. Ideas of good parenting, for example, will be value-laden and aspirationally and culturally sensitive and not necessarily directly informed by systematic research. This makes ideas about good parenting suitable subjects for discussion and exploration of points of view. The partnership model requires knowledge about the groups and individuals that constitute the target audience for the programme, and an understanding of their objectives, for it is only on the basis of such knowledge that those authentic exchanges that form a basis for enhanced or altered awareness can take place.

Traditionally, those engaged in adult education have been encouraged to think about characteristics of adult learners in terms of what it is that makes adults special as participants in formal educational activities. We can start to reflect upon this simply by considering the differences between adults and children (though care must be taken not to exaggerate the differences: children are also individuals). An obvious point is that adults have lived longer than children. This rather uninteresting, or very obvious, fact has a number of very significant implications.

First, as a result of living longer, the learner has a substantial body of experience upon which to draw. Experience provides an opportunity for engagement. Experience has both positive and negative aspects when considered in relation to formal learning. The positive aspect of experience is that it means that adults have something to contribute to their own and to each other's learning. In this sense, any teaching method or curriculum design process that calls for the specification and application of this experience can only add to the richness of what takes place on a programme or within a given session.

A negative aspect is that an individual's experience may be limited or tending towards inappropriate conclusions. If we have lived a long time, our experience may be valuable in some ways, but a hindrance in others, and we only really become aware of this when challenged by new contexts, such as encountering specific applications of the rapid developments in information technology or talking with new people. Someone with considerable experience of labour markets and labour market expectations from the past may face problems in trying to understand the behaviour and expectations of younger people who are faced with a radically different set of circumstances. Adult learners can feel a loss of status in coming to terms with adjusting their expectations and understanding in the light of new contexts and of other people's experiences. Where experience is to be challenged, the diversity of experience in a group can offer safe ways of doing this provided that trust and sensitivity are developed early on within the group. Either way, if the programme can engage with the individual and group experience, then learning activities are more likely to be successful from everyone's point of view.

Second, because adult learners have something to gain and something to lose in the context of a programme, the dignity of the learner is something that has to be reflected upon. This is the case at all levels of education – respect for children and young people is also important in schooling. Participants hope to gain skills and knowledge (the key learning outcomes in curriculum development terms, as specified in the publicity and course details) otherwise they would not have opted for the particular programme of study. They may become irritated if they do not gain such skills. In addition, they may also hope to experience a sense of development by being part of a group with similar interests or sharing similar hopes and fears. Both aspects will be of particular importance in birth and parenthood classes. However, an aspect of adult learning is that it is normally non-compulsory and this gives an added dimension. People can, and often do, vote with their feet and leave if the delivery and content do not match their expectations. The programme needs to address both cognitive and affective aspects; in other words, the experience has to work educationally and rationally as well as socially and emotionally. So those responsible for delivery could think of themselves, for example, as good hosts who make sure that participants are comfortable with all aspects of the social interactions in the session; guides who help shape the knowledge, and help develop a route plan so that participants know where they are and why they are engaging in the given activities; and motivators, helping participants see what they have achieved thus far and how they have grown during the programme. If participants are not provided with a safe environment in which to contribute, take risks and grow, then they may feel that their status is diminished or that the risks are too high and simply withdraw.

The theoretical insight that is helpful to consider here is Maslow's hierarchy of needs.

Abraham Maslow rejected a Freudian approach to the study of human psychology. Whereas Freud studied those exhibiting mental ill-health, Maslow felt that a study of the fully functioning healthy individual would give rise to useful insights into human motivation. So he opted to look at people operating in situations of affection and playfulness or those whose lives were fulfilled – think of a possible example of such an emotionally healthy person from amongst the range of people that you know. Maslow felt that healthy people were basically reliable (exhibiting authentic behaviour and all that this implies), self-protecting and self-regulating. In other words, he held a benevolent view of fulfilled human nature. This may seem at odds

Figure 2.1
Maslow's hierarchy of needs

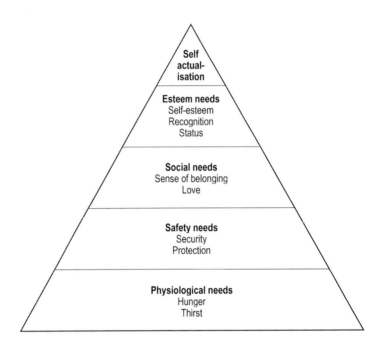

with historical or more recent experience: people fight wars and engage in brutality. These events have occurred throughout history but the whole of human history is not simply about wars and brutality. Most of the time, people are getting on with each other and we all rely on the cooperation and goodwill of others in order to get through each day. It is a normal expectation of traffic flows that traffic will be orderly as a result of orderly and cooperative behaviour (think of drivers being able to pull out of side roads onto busy main roads as a result of cooperative behaviour from other drivers). Maslow is not alone in thinking that human nature is essentially benevolent. There is a tradition supporting such a view that goes back to the first decades of the 18th century, and to a Scottish philosopher called Francis Hutcheson. Maslow's insight was that violent and disruptive behaviour only occurs because the hierarchy of needs has not been fulfilled and as a consequence human nature is frustrated in its drive towards benevolence. A result of unfulfilled lower level needs is selfish behaviour. Self*less* behaviour is the result of lower-level 'deficiencies' being filled.

At a basic level we need to have bodily needs satisfied. If these are not satisfied, irritation and sickness is the result. To move on, the bodily needs need to be satisfied. Safety needs come next. We all require a place to feel secure in, such as a loving family or a supportive group. At the next level there is the need to belong in a wider world, to be part of a bigger group at work or in clubs or in religious organisations. The need for esteem comes next. Esteem can come from being a competent individual, recognised as such by the self and also by others. If all these lower needs are satisfied then individuals can aspire to 'self-actualisation'. This is not strictly a need but a state of being in which people become more and more themselves, realising their full human potential. If lower level needs are a source of frustration because they are not being met, then the chances of achieving self-actualisation are slim. But Maslow's message to adult educators must be that given an education that is capable of assisting people to grow and develop, by being positive and joyful, we can all move towards self-actualisation. This means thinking through ways by which we can enhance the confidence of participants by giving them a sense of participation in and ownership of their own learning.

Whilst Maslow is concerned with the big issues of human psychology, his ideas can be used to think through simple issues with respect to a programme of study. It is not inappropriate to reflect on participants' needs in a similar way. Maslow's hierarchy reminds us to think about issues such as how people *feel*, rather than simply concentrating on subject-expertise or upon knowledge to be developed. One way of doing this is by asking such questions as will help us develop our role as educators. In course planning, the following can be useful prompts:

- What steps have we taken to ensure that people are comfortable and that there are clean toilets and that refreshments are available?
- Is the teaching environment warm and properly ventilated?
- What steps can we take to ensure that the individuals who come to a class are helped to be part of a purposeful and constructive group?
- How can we encourage and reward participants so that they feel confident about what they are doing?
- Can we help participants get it right – and what do we do if they do not?

Sensitive answers to such questions help promote the partnership approach to learning.

A third implication of the fact that adults have lived longer than young people, is that each person has taken a particular path through life and in a modern market-oriented economy, that path will have made possible greater degrees of specialisation and diversity than in the past. The participants will have some experiences in common and many that are diverse. A context of cultural diversity will also give rise to situations where there are some experiences in common and others that are qualitatively different. So any educator who is interested in working in partnership with a group is likely to find that it is useful to reflect on the diversity of experience that adults bring to a class. This can only be done, at the planning stage, by thinking about adults in general or, at a less abstract level, reflecting on the kinds of people who have come to the class in the past and the contexts within which they have operated.

But the problem is that in any kind of learning and teaching, we do not work with, and can never work with, 'adults in general'. Indeed, there is a sense in which this notion can lead to idealisation at best and stereotyping at worst. We can only work with the particular group of people that have been prepared to enrol on our programme. This group will be composed of people with differing backgrounds, aspirations and experiences. To gain insight into what motivates the group in the context of the programme, it is useful to have a set of activities or an approach to the curriculum that gives us a chance to understand the context and aspirations of the particular set of individuals that make up the class. Participants are trying to achieve something. By attending, they are opting for some sort of change in understanding or some sort of intellectual and emotional growth. If we are to help them learn, it is useful to have an indication of what it is they are trying to achieve. This means some carefully selected icebreaker exercises or group-building activities or simple hopes/fears exercises that will help create the group and provide information on individuals. It also means that we need to be prepared to create opportunities for discussion. Discussion can lead to some surprising and creative outcomes. Opportunities to talk over aspects of the curriculum first in pairs, then in small groups and finally in one large group will help promote the right kind of social context for learning by building relationships and confidence, and so help to secure group and individual ownership of the learning.

One implication of diversity is that mature people come to programmes with different approaches to learning. Adult education literature has always recognised that different people learn in different ways. This is partly determined by experience and partly by preferences. Some older people may feel uncomfortable with group work and discussion because they have had an experience of education that has been about sitting in rows and only making limited contributions. Any resistance is usually easily overcome by making people feel comfortable and easing in the new method. Midwives and parenthood educators are not likely to face this problem directly – the typical participant is a younger rather than an older adult – but at least the example points out that sometimes teaching and learning methods may need to be gently socialised. Again, it is well-documented in the established literature that some people prefer to grasp problems intuitively, others wish to work through the logic to promote their understanding; some need lots of concrete examples whilst others can move to abstract ideas and principles very quickly. Since we cannot be certain in advance of the composition of any group with respect to their preferences in learning, then common sense suggests an approach to the planning of the learning and teaching that allows for a range of ways of participating, e.g. some listening, some watching, some discussion; some practical work; some reflection; some theory; some small group discussion and some large group discussion, and so on.

What switches people 'off'?

We have had a look at what switches people on to learning. It is worthwhile thinking through what switches people off, but only to give us a guide as to what to avoid. Knowing what switches people on to learning is likely to be sufficient to lead towards good outcomes. In general terms a closed, unidirectional, expert-based method of delivery will not get the best response from participants, except in closely defined circumstances. Positive adult learning calls for activity, diversity of methods, discussion and social interaction and a growing sense of independence within a supporting social environment. Such an environment creates a sense of movement and growth. Tapping into the individual and group experience helps create links with past learning or to give the curriculum direct relevance and meaning to people. A negative environment for learning will be created by approaches that encourage passivity rather than action and where the teacher owns all aspects of the curriculum. Where little attention is paid to the group and the individuals who make it up, there will tend to be low commitment and dwindling attendance. Passivity and isolation will constitute the social experience and a culture of dependence will be in place. In an active class it is the participants who will be carrying most of the work and the teacher will be helping to 'shape' the learning.

LEARNING STYLES: MODELS AND IMPLICATIONS

In the context of a labour-expensive market economy, most of us have come across flat-pack furniture, at some stage, and we may even have come across a range of experiences relating to the assembly of flat-packed furniture. It is clear that there are many different approaches to building an item. One person may prefer a systematic approach, reading all the information, setting out the various large and small pieces in order, checking the items against the inventory and then assembling the furniture by strictly following the instructions in a linear way. A second person may prefer to have a go, by trial and error, applying experience from other related activities or sensing a way towards the object as a whole. A third person may move between the two methods, sometimes following instructions, sometimes proceeding by trial and error. Talk about different learning styles is pointing to the phenomenon – exemplified by the three (fictional) characters in the story that has just been told – that people approach learning tasks in different ways. This is the case both for practical activity, such as assembling flat-packed furniture, and for academic activities. We are not all the same, even when it comes to engaging in our own learning.

There are now many formal ways of trying to identify learning styles. In the next section, a brief account of the Kolb Learning Style Inventory will be given.

Kolb Learning Inventory

The Kolb Learning Inventory (KLI) makes a four-fold division of learning styles. The inventory is easy to use and requires no special training: learners rate themselves according to a simple set of choices offered in terms of simple attributes (this is a weakness as well as a strength). The KLI emerged from a longer intellectual development built around the notion of experiential learning, an idea that draws intellectual justification from the works of educational philosophers such as Dewey, Lewin and Piaget as well as others. Individuals, when it comes to absorbing information, may have a preference for either 'concrete experience' (doing something, or making something, or touching something, or changing something) or 'abstract conceptualisation' (coming at it through theory and thought rather than through feelings). When it comes to making the ideas their own, individuals will have preferences between 'active experimentation' (trying ideas out and seeing if they work) and 'reflective organisation' (watching and thinking).

The Kolb Learning Inventory is used to map individuals into a grid that has four dimensions. These dimensions are built around experience, reflection, theoretical understanding and action. The sequence when set out in an ordered and circular diagram is known as the Kolb Learning Cycle. This has been popularised in a number of ways as adult educators searched for simpler ways of working with their own participants within the general methodology of experiential learning; experience has been characterised as 'doing', reflection as 'reviewing' or even 'talking', abstract conceptualisation as 'thinking' or 'generalising' and 'active experimentation' as 'action' or 'action and change'.

As there are two sets of paired choices, there are, according to the Learning Style Inventory, four types of learners. Each of these types engages in learning from different perspectives. The categories are set out in Kolb's work, from which the following is derived.

Type one: concrete, reflective

These learners are interested in outcomes and so are looking for motivation. Such learners will be concerned with questions such as: 'Why are we doing this?' 'What are the outcomes likely to be?' 'How

Figure 2.2
Diagram of the Kolb Learning
Cycle

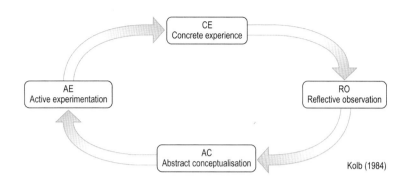

Kolb (1984)

does it relate to my experience?' The tutor works best with such students as a motivator, helping them link ideas to experience. Relevance and application are the key motivators for such learners.

Type two: abstract, reflective

This type of learner responds well to systematically presented information, i.e. ideas and knowledge presented in a structured way such as lectures and presentations. This type of learner tends to ask questions such as: 'What are we being asked to learn?' 'What are the implications?' The tutor is likely to be able to work with such students as a reliable subject-expert who delivers logical and systematic information. Such learners respond well to formally organised and structured presentations.

Type three: abstract, active

An appreciation of problem-focused learning with some limited experimentation and (carefully-managed) risk-taking characterises this type of learner. It helps if the problems in which they are engaged are well-defined. The relationship between tutors and such learners may be best thought of as that of coaching. The tutor as coach retains the role of expert. For this kind of learner, bounded practice is of major significance.

Type four: concrete, active

This type of learner appreciates the opportunity to apply new knowledge to authentic and problematic situations. Set up situations for such learners with open-ended tasks in which there is the possibility of discovery leading to new applications. Such learners tend to be interested in asking speculative or experimental questions such as 'What would happen if ...?', though in a context of action and change. Successful relationships between students and teacher should be like mentoring, where the teacher is encouraging growth, rather than coaching.

A principal aim of identifying learning styles is to help learners understand their own strengths and weaknesses with respect to how they go about learning. Experiencing the cycle is meant to help adjust the learner to be open to new ways of learning. It is hoped that someone armed with this knowledge and engaged in a variety of educational activities and experiences will develop as an independent, self-directed and self-actualising learner. Someone who likes to do practical tasks is likely to feel uncomfortable when called upon to reflect. If this is the case, when free to choose, such a person will choose tasks over reflection and socially avoid the other experience. The Kolb approach suggests that this is a social preference and so we should not assume that such preferences are fixed for all time. Activists can learn to reflect or at least to benefit from the reflections of others, and so on. It is clear that carefully selected group work will make it possible for learners to experience the whole cycle as each member is drawn into a relationship with those who are likely to have a different approach.

So if we are trying to reach all participants, it is a good idea to know some of the implications of the learning styles, even if we may not be in a position to be able to analyse particular groups. A unidirectional lecture or a very formal presentation will only easily engage type two learners (abstract, reflective) but for the other types it would be a rather unsuccessful experience. A well thought out programme of study will move the whole group around the cycle in carefully selected ways.

A benefit that arises from the Kolb Learning Inventory and the related Kolb Learning Cycle is that it can be used to construct an experiential curriculum which 'touches' all aspects relevant to the educational progress of adults: experience, reflection, generalisation, action and change. From the point of view of learning, no part of the cycle is privileged. Think of a wheel. It is hard to talk about the circumference as having a privileged part, for one bit touches the ground after another in rapid succession. It only works because this is the case. So in the Kolb Learning Cycle no particular approach is any better than any other. For full and complete learning, all parts of the cycle need to be experienced. This is one of the reasons that we work in mixed groups: so that problems can be explored from different points of view. The section that follows will explore the 'curriculum' uses of the Kolb Learning Cycle.

Using Kolb to think about curriculum design

A central idea in working with the Kolb model as a possible curriculum model is the process that it takes participants through. It allows participants to experience all aspects of the cycle, even bits where they as individuals may experience a 'bumpy ride'. The approach to learning styles suggested by Kolb is that they are preferences but not fixed in stone. Action-oriented learners can come to appreciate the contribution that reflection can make, even if they feel less comfortable with reflection. Using Kolb as a way of thinking about a curriculum (or bits of a curriculum) is one way of ensuring that all get to participate in a way that suits them and learn that the whole cycle is needed for fully developed learning.

Experience

This can be brought in from outside or created by exercises within the programme. Accessing experience helps give the group a context, in relation to the programme, to each other and to their own learning needs. Tapping experience does not have to be daunting. Asking participants to make a list of the five key questions that they would like to see explored in the programme can help check the relevance of what is on offer and so shape some negotiation. Asking participants to compare one list with that of another person and seeing if there are things in common, can initiate useful and non-threatening discussion. Getting feedback from the whole group, with points noted on a flip-chart, and seeing if and how the planned agenda can accommodate diversity, can further the required negotiations. It can also help the tutor gauge the level of experience in the group and the resources within the group that can be drawn upon to enhance the learning of other participants. Keeping the flip-chart list for use at the end of the programme, as part of the session aimed at closure, can help illustrate what has been covered and so provide a basis for monitoring the progress made.

Reflection

This usually involves discussion with others. Paired discussion is a useful starting point where issues are sensitive or where the group is only just forming. It is sometimes useful to encourage participants to work with someone new to them. Comparing experiences and highlighting points that are similar and points that are different is a useful way of developing a reflective capacity. Reflection helps to make overt feelings or ideas that were covert and so difficult to specify, monitor or change.

Generalisation

This is where a set of principles is extracted from the experience and reflection. This is often a whole-group discussion and guided by the tutor. It is at this stage that the group gives 'meaning' to the experiences and discussion. Any theoretical insight from the group can be supplemented, where gaps exist, by subject knowledge.

Action and change

This is where individuals think through the consequences of what they have experienced. Sometimes the statements are about change and sometimes they are about affirmation; either way, at this stage individuals are encouraged to say what the experience or the learning means to them. Have the starting point questions and behaviours been modified? Has a better set of values or questions been discovered? Individuals are expected at this stage to monitor their own learning.

This is done by identifying for themselves what has been learned and by working out the implications that result. An interesting exercise in programme closure is to get a list of what has been learned by taking contributions from each participant (one point from each around the room until all points have been exhausted).

Although the notion of learning styles is useful, particularly as a description or organiser of ideas about learning styles, it is important not to give any particular means of identifying learning styles an intellectual weight that it cannot carry. The Kolb Learning Cycle and associated inventory comes out of a serious intellectual tradition but it can be criticised as too simple or lacking a notion of conflict that some would see as important in the development of learning theory or of being unreliable as people learn to second-guess the questions. It has been used here in a 'potted' version as a means of shaping a discussion about linking the notion of a diversity of adult learners to notions of a diversity of approaches to learning and teaching activities. It is descriptively useful in this context but it is not the only means of identifying learning styles.

CONCLUDING REMARKS

The main aim of this chapter has been to provide perspectives on the contexts that adult learners bring to participation in a programme of study and the implications and challenges that these can create for those interested in providing learning and teaching opportunities for adult students. The key ideas are essentially simple. Adults learn best when their experiences are acknowledged and challenged; when attention is paid to the social context of the learning; when there is an emphasis on confidence building, growth, generating a sense of direction and ownership and when risk-taking is encouraged in an atmosphere of trust and understanding. The aim is to help participants develop as independent, self-confident learners through engaging in a variety of ways in the curriculum. While we can derive insight into the learning and teaching process from a reflection upon adults in general, we can only work with the particular group of participants who come along to our programmes. This means we need to translate those general insights into action to get to know people as individuals and help shape them into a group that can promote each other's learning. It is easier to do this if we ourselves are prepared to adopt a reflective approach to our own learning and to that of others. Taking care of social needs by reflecting upon Maslow and taking care of individual preferences in learning by reflecting upon the implications of different learning styles can also help mediate between the knowledge and learning and teaching processes. How to do this better within the context of antenatal education is the subject matter of the rest of this book.

FURTHER READING

Brown M, Fry H, Marshall S 1999 Reflective practice. In: Fry H, Ketteridge K, Marshall M (eds) A Handbook for Teaching and Learning in Higher Education. Kogan Page, London, p 207-219

Boud D, Miller N 1996 Working with experience: animating learning. Routledge, London

Burnard P 1990 Learning human skills: an experiential guide for nurses. Heineman Nursing, Oxford

Corder N 2002 Learning to teach adults. Routledge, London

Dennison W F 1990 Do, review, learn, apply: a simple guide to experiential learning. Blackwell Education, Oxford

Gibbs G 1988 Learning by doing: a guide to teaching and learning methods. FEU, London

Honey P 2000 Learning log: a way to enhance learning from experience. Peter Honey Publications, Maidenhead.

Honey P, Mumford A 1989 The manual of learning opportunities. Peter Honey Publications, Maidenhead

Kolb D A 1976 The Learning Style Inventory: Technical manual. McBer, Boston, Massachussetts

Kolb D A 1984 Experiential learning. Prentice Hall, Englewood Cliffs, New Jersey

Knowles M S 1990 The adult learner: a neglected species, 4th edn. Gulf Publishing Co., London

Maslow A H 1968 Towards a psychology of being. Van Nostrad Reinhold, New York

Schön D 1987 Educating the reflective practitioner. Jossey-Bass, San Francisco

Chapter 3

Why Education for Birth is Important

Alexandra Smith

In view of the fact that intervention in labour seems to be increasing, with caesarean section rates now approaching 25% nationally, and normal birth on the decline, is there any point in committing to education for birth? If the environment of birth is so hostile to parents putting into practice the skills they have learned in antenatal classes, and to implementing the decisions about intervention and pain relief which they had hoped to make, is childbirth education a waste of time? It may be that outcome measures are not all that counts when considering the effectiveness of antenatal education, and that the process of an educational encounter based on respect for the autonomy and lived experiences of expectant parents yields its own rewards, though these are more difficult to measure than epidural uptake or forceps rates.

(Editors' note)

Those of us who run antenatal classes will often be asked what they are about. It is not always easy to give a succinct answer. At different times we have tried to sum up the ethos of a particular approach in a single pithy phrase such as 'Informed Choice' or 'Preparation for Parenthood' but these concepts are so tantalisingly loaded that they have become excellent openers for a debate rather than simple explanations of purpose. However, in order to measure and affirm the importance of our work as childbirth educators, especially at this time when childbirth is in crisis, we do need to be aware of exactly what it is we are hoping to achieve, how we hope to achieve this, and what might get in the way.

LEARNING AIMS AND OUTCOMES

To assist in the evaluation process, good teachers establish clear aims and learning outcomes, and develop strategies or approaches designed to meet these. If effective, these strategies will enable learning to take place and people will be able to:

- Do something new or better than before
- Know something they didn't know before
- Feel, believe or understand something with greater depth or insight
- And, very importantly, make use of the new skill, knowledge or understanding.

But will this learning be of any importance? It is quite possible that I may be very good at teaching something that, in the grand scheme of things, doesn't really matter.

For example (and please transpose a childbirth issue of your choice onto the following analogy …) my grape peeling lessons are very successful. The teaching methods I use are clearly effective because, by the end of the course, everyone can peel grapes beautifully – but are peeled grapes really important? If not, then neither are the grape-peeling lessons. The importance of learning is measured by the degree of impact that the learning has on the life of a particular individual or group of individuals, whether they are conscious of this or not.

There is another way of looking at this though – a way in which the grape peeling lessons may still have importance despite the fact that we attach very little social or cultural significance to peeled grapes. That is that *process* may be more important than *product*.

Process and product

The product is *what* you are hoping the people in your class will learn. The process is *how* you are helping them to learn it.

Your intended learning product is usually expressed as a series of learning outcomes. These are based on the acquisition of knowledge, skills and understanding specific to the content or subject matter of the class.

If we were to measure the importance of grape peeling classes in terms of how often the learning product (in this case, the ability to peel a grape) is put to later use and the impact it has on the person's life, we may have to conclude that the learning has not been very important. The person may have discovered that they have no real interest in grape peeling after all. Or they may have arrived at the belief that grape peel is good for you. On the other hand there may exist some socio-economic or political restraint that makes grape peeling very difficult or impossible. For example, an embargo on the importation of grapes at the time would thwart the most ardent enthusiast. Or a strong cultural or familial disbelief in the practice would prevent all but the most assertive people from getting their grape-peelers out. And then there may be environmental barriers to using the skill freely. I for one don't feel at home peeling grapes in someone else's kitchen, particularly if they insist on watching me closely with a critical eye or I am pushed for time. These and similar restraints may influence the potential importance of what was learnt in the class. It has not been possible to put learning into practice. Therefore it is not possible to measure its importance.

One other major consideration to bear in mind when assessing the importance of the learning experience is the distance in time between the learning and the assessment. Situations change and over time a person may, for a number of reasons, find that they are able to put past learning into practice, or that it has meaning for them for the first time, long after it was initially evaluated as being unimportant. The learning may have been a vital piece of a jigsaw that wasn't completed until much later.

So, product-based learning may:

- Be unimportant at the end of the day
- Have its potential importance frustrated or blocked
- Be stored in a 'keep until needed' file and not recognised as having importance until much later
- Or be important straight away – in that it makes an immediate and significant impact in the life of an individual or group of individuals.

Returning to process – how may the way in which the learning outcomes were reached have importance too?

> The purpose of instruction is to transfer knowledge and expertise. It is based on methods of learning. Education, on the other hand, aims to awaken and develop faculties which are latent in the individual, involving physical, emotional, intellectual, moral and spiritual aspects. So education can be defined as 'the implementation of methods which allow a human being to take shape and develop.'
> (Bertin, 2003)

In my grape peeling classes I deliberately use a range of strategies or teaching methods that help people learn (Robertson, 1999). As with other practical skills, grape peeling is not really something you can learn to do by listening to someone talking about it – or even by watching a demonstration. Therefore I use lots of interactive approaches.

My process strategies include:

- Problem solving activities
- Discussion
- Group projects

In the process I also:

- Listen to people
- Value and utilise existing knowledge and skills
- Appreciate other people's

- Working in pairs
- Design and planning
- Creative opportunities
- Student presentations
- Practice and experimentation
- And lots of laughter

insights
- Give praise and encouragement
- Show respect
- Show interest
- Create a setting in which people behave this way toward each other

This process will hopefully make it easier for people to achieve the product-based learning outcomes. It may also result in another kind of learning that is incidental to the primary objectives of the course. This secondary learning could have immense importance that goes unrecognised and therefore unmeasured. For example, I am surprised by the number of people on my grape peeling course who, after a few weeks, find themselves initiating major transformations in their lives. Some discover they now have the confidence to go onto further study of another sort, others embark on career developments, close personal relationships change, and many long-lasting and significant friendships are made. Learning has been a catalyst for change in ways that could not be planned for and are difficult to measure. If nothing else, the laughter alone has proven health benefits (Berk & Stanley, 1996).

To summarise:

- Process based learning outcomes such as increased confidence and self-esteem help learners make use of their new skills, knowledge or understanding.

But the importance of process-based learning is difficult to measure because:

- The learning may be transferred to other situations and not put into effect in the expected setting.
- The learner may feel that the change has come from within and not attribute it to the learning event. This should nonetheless be a great boost to the teacher's ego because enabling a person to access their innate strengths is true empowerment.

THE INFLUENCE OF THE TEACHER

Even when learning outcomes are achieved (that is, at the end of the course people demonstrate new knowledge, skills and insight) it may not be possible to put the learning into use (see Figure 3.5). If learning is not used it cannot make a difference to what subsequently happens. If there is no difference in what happens the learning will be assessed as being unimportant.

> *Research evaluated the use of the whole set of MIDIRS Informed Choice leaflets across maternity units to assess their effectiveness in promoting informed choice. Between 92% and 99% of women who received each leaflet reported that it was helpful or very helpful. However, there was no evidence that the leaflets were effective in increasing the proportion of women who reported having exercised informed choice.*
> (Kirkham & Stapleton, 2001)

The information in the MIDIRS leaflets was not sufficient in itself to enable women to use what they learned to bring about change. Is it possible that the attitudes of the midwives sharing this information, in their role as antenatal educators, may have been influential in this?

Which of these antenatal teachers do you most closely resemble?

- Dorothy tells women what to expect. She is a messenger for 'the system'. Secretly she is quite afraid of birth but hopes that her fear doesn't show. Dorothy gives a series of talks about the different topics and welcomes questions.
- Paula tells women what they should do. She is a promoter for a cause. Paula has strong views that she believes passionately in. Her classes are very lively but she has a tendency to sermonise.
- Sarah enables women to identify and meet their own particular needs. She is a facilitator, enabler, advocate and friend. She is an excellent and non-judgemental listener and responds to the individual needs of her group with a variety of learning strategies.

Most of us are probably a complicated blend of all three. We have our secret fears, and our duties to other bodies – and we have our passions and our professionalism. The Dorothy in us is concerned with telling women about the 'reality' of the situation. She knows that most women give birth in hospital and in reality over 1 in 5 will have a caesarean. The Paula in us wants women to know how it could be – that most women could safely give birth at home and 98% of women could breastfeed. Our inner Sarah is, in theory, the model antenatal teacher. Unlike Dorothy and Paula, she is not didactic. She believes in informed choice and she understands that for learning to be important it has to be matched to the needs of the learner – it has to be relevant and important to them.

In practice, Sarah and Paula can encounter problems in the way they teach. For example, when Sarah gives impartial, research-based information about pethidine she is sometimes accused of being anti-drugs. She is seen as having donned her Paula persona. She does not want to be seen this way and consequently may fall into the 'three advantages of pethidine and three disadvantages of pethidine' trap where, in her need to appear to be objective, she distorts information that is clearly weighted one way, to make it seem balanced. Paula, on the other hand, can be very inspiring. She can open people's eyes. Her strength of conviction is infectious. It can enable women to discover their own strength and make real changes. But these changes sometimes involve 'non-compliance' and Paula is then stigmatised as a troublemaker or an extremist by some of her peers. Even though her convictions are sound, parents may be led by others to mistrust her. But Dorothy doesn't have these problems. She toes the party line. She doesn't want women to worry unnecessarily or be set up for disappointment, so she provides carefully selected and approved information aimed at allaying fears and encouraging women to trust the experts who are caring for them. Being Dorothy feels safe but is not empowering, either for herself or for those she teaches.

Beliefs about the intrinsic importance of the birth experience – does one day matter?

Dorothy feels that birth is only 'one day' and that as long as mother and baby are well that is all that matters. But Paula believes that giving birth is a unique and formative experience. It may only be one day, but it is a critical day – a crisis in the true meaning of the word, a turning point, and a rite of passage. A woman remembers the details of each birth for the rest of her life (Simkin, 1992). Whether she felt strong and capable or overpowered and helpless – these feelings will have remained to help form the way she sees herself as a person (Peterson, 1996; Hodnett, 2002). Therefore, the nature of the birth experience is immensely important. This is true not only for the mother but for the baby too – perhaps in ways we do not yet fully understand.

> *Anyone present at a birth is bound to be deeply disturbed ... no doubt this is because we have all experienced birth. There are echoes of it deep inside us, as powerful as they are suppressed. Nothing is forgotten – birth least of all.*
> (Leboyer, 1975:95)
>
> *Childbirth ... presents to women a unique and powerful opportunity to find their core strength in a manner that forever changes their self-perception. Additionally, it can offer women an experience in trusting their body wisdom in a way that may alter how they respond throughout life to health challenges.*
> (Nichols & Humenick, 2000:xiii)

Kate is awaiting the arrival of her first baby. She has vague fears about the birth but tries not to dwell on them. She just wants to get the ordeal out of the way. She feels there is nothing she can realistically do to make a difference to what happens anyway. Kate wants as normal and as safe a birth as possible so she puts herself into the best hands (at

Figure 3.1
A vicious circle
(with thanks to Niamh Healy)

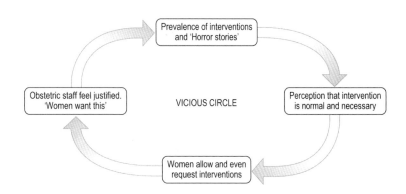

a consultant hospital) and adopts Dorothy's attitude as a positive way of subduing disquiet – 'it's only one day'. She feels this is a good philosophy and a valid coping mechanism. Kate may be lucky and have a very positive birthing experience but in reality her chances of having that normal birth in hospital are dwindling year by year. Kate doesn't know this and Dorothy certainly hasn't told her – she doesn't want to rock the boat. Paula thinks this is very wrong. Without that knowledge, Kate is unknowingly submitting to attitudes of care that may well confirm her worst fears about birth.

She has become part of a vicious circle where intervention is 'the new normal' – and where women's fear is 'cured' by ever increasing amounts of medicine and surgery.

Paula believes that education for birth is vital in order to counteract the prevailing climate of fear. She agrees with independent midwife Tricia Anderson's sentiments that childbirth is in crisis, women need to be told the truth and childbirth educators and midwives *should* be rocking the boat (Anderson 2003).

Sarah sometimes wonders if Paula is allowing her personal feelings too long a leash. Paula argues that, equally, it is personal motives that lead many teachers to deliberately or unconsciously withhold information – and in consequence, women unwittingly comply, even collude, with a system that is becoming increasingly medicalised and, very often, not in their best interests.

The medicalisation of birth

These are some of the things that Paula thinks Kate needs to know the truth about:

- The overall caesarean section rate in England and Wales has risen from 4% in 1970 to 21.5% (Thomas & Paranjothy, 2001). The World Health Organization reports that there is no improvement in outcome after 8% (Henderson, 2002) and recommends the rate should be no higher than 10 – 15% as in Denmark, Norway and Sweden (Parliamentary Office of Science and Technology, 2002).

- Caesarean section significantly increases maternal mortality and morbidity (Waterstone, Bewley, Wolfe 2001) and results in lower levels of maternal satisfaction (Miller, Thornton & Gittens, 2002).
- Since 1992, the percentage of women experiencing a normal birth has declined from 57.2% to 44.4% (National Childbirth Trust, 2002).
- A recent study on home birth compared the results of 4,600 (largely low-risk) women who planned a home birth with 3,300 equivalent women who planned a hospital birth. Women who planned a hospital birth were twice as likely to have a forceps or ventouse delivery, or a caesarean delivery, than those who planned a home birth (Chamberlain, Wraight, Crowley 1997).
- Home birth is at least as safe as hospital birth for women with uncomplicated pregnancies (Young, Hey, 2000) – and possibly safer. It has been estimated that in Britain over 3,000 babies die each year as a direct result of their mothers choosing to give birth in hospital (Beech, 2000).
- 10% of all patients admitted to British hospitals experience an adverse event, about half of which are preventable (Vincent & Neale, 2001).

Without this knowledge, Kate is disadvantaged. If she does not know that there are implications from following a medical approach to maternity care – implications that may work against her chances of experiencing a normal birth – she will not be sufficiently motivated to pursue alternatives. And if she does not know there are alternatives – she is powerless.

Institutionalisation of birth

Even when we are familiar with it, the sort of information above can be hard to swallow. It is easy to believe that hospital is the normal place

Figure 3.2
The institutionalisation of birth

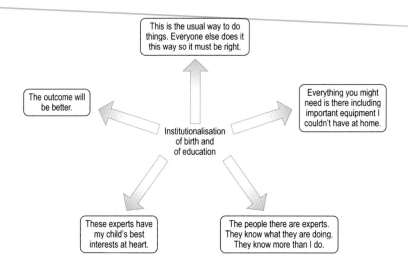

to have babies because it is easy to see that this is where most babies are born. This is where the problem lies. Free and equal access to health care for all pregnant women (considered to be a good thing) takes some organising. Prevailing logic leads to this operating in a central and public place. But in this institutional environment it is hard to individualise care and birth has become a medical event. (And many consider this a bad thing.) By agreeing to the good part we hand over power to the organisers and, in our powerlessness, helplessly accept the bad part – very quickly accepting it as normal. The same has happened with the institutionalisation of education. Arguments to support both institutions are identical and equally questionable.

What we see is institutionalised birth – not elemental birth. Few people today, particularly obstetricians, will ever see the normality of birth within the home and therefore cannot conceive this to be possible. It is unthinkable – and if something is unthinkable it cannot be an option when making decisions.

PERSONAL CONSTRUCTS

We create the realities that govern our decision making from what we know and what we can see. Constructivism in psychology holds that learners construct new ideas or concepts based upon their current or past knowledge. When a person is called upon to construct ideas about a novel occurrence, for example, the imminent birth of a first child, the recognition of partial similarity with a known experience provides the basis for analogy. The learner selects and transforms information, constructs hypotheses, and makes decisions, relying on a cognitive structure to do so (Botella, 2003).

Kate, who we met earlier, might offer an example:

- Kate needs to construct new ideas. She hasn't given birth before so she is not sure what to think.
- She transforms information she already has from situations that seem similar to her. She sees that birth almost always happens in hospital settings and it looks a bit like an operation. This is her analogy.
- She constructs a hypothesis. She supposes that, if it is a bit like an operation, it must be quite dangerous and something best left to the experts.
- And arrives at a decision. She decides to have her baby in hospital as well.

Kate chooses hospital birth by default because, in her reality, there is no other course of action open to her.

'By default' is defined by Chambers (1995) as a course of action taken when no specific alternative instruction is given or because of someone's failure to do something that would have prevented or altered the situation.

Figure 3.3
A virtuous circle

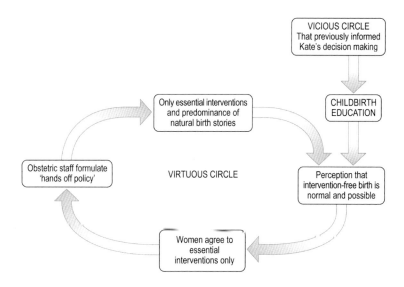

Making a decision by default is not informed choice. Women do not actively choose to have hospital births or epidurals or caesarean sections – not in the same way as we might say, 'Coffee cake? Chocolate cake? Mmm, I think I'll go for the Coffee.'

Women resort to these things because the alternatives:

- Are not offered at all.
- Are not offered with the same enthusiasm or with the same support.
- Are unimaginable – so rarely encountered that they are hard to picture. 'I can't see myself doing that.'
- Threaten the woman's sense of security in belonging to the mainstream group.

This is where childbirth education can intervene in important ways. Childbirth education can promote a virtuous circle by intervening at the second stage of Kate's cognitive process and helping her to construct the perception that intervention-free birth is normal and possible – that birth is a physiological process that her body is capable of – and not a bit like an operation at all.

IF BIRTH IS A NORMAL PHYSIOLOGICAL PROCESS – WHY DO WE NEED TO TEACH ABOUT IT?

If we really believe that birth is a normal physiological process and if we really believe that women have all the knowledge and resources within them that they will need – then the idea of education does seem unnecessary. It could be likened to teaching a community about digestion. If the way of life in this community is such that almost everyone has perfect digestion, there will be little need to hold digestion education classes. If, however, the pattern of life changes in this idyll, life becomes more stressful, meals are rushed, new ideas about food are introduced, home cooking declines as more and more the art of cuisine and the science of nutrition enter the realm of a select group of specialists, and frequent indigestion becomes accepted as normal – then education, or re-education, would seem to be called for.

To restore optimum levels of normality the focus for the classes that Paula would run would not be on normal digestion (she believes the potential for this is already in place). Instead she would focus on helping people to recognise that frequent indigestion is not normal or necessary but very often the result of cultural and social disturbance to the natural processes. If these disturbances are truly addressed, normality resumes.

Dorothy would be quite concerned about digestion education classes with this focus. She herself does not feel equal to challenging the new order of things so it is likely that many of the course participants will feel the same. She worries they will leave the classes still eating in the same way but feeling guiltier about it. So Dorothy feels more comfortable working from within the new order and offering information about 'making the most of eating out' and 'different menus on offer'.

Similarly, the majority of childbirth education classes have the major focus on aspects of birth that do not happen spontaneously and from within but rather those that are instigated by others and are done to the woman – occasionally vital but widely accepted or tolerated because of the cultural warping of our expectations. Items on the class agenda may include for example:

- When you go for your scan
- Routine induction
- When to go to hospital
- What happens on arrival
- Coping with internals
- Pharmaceutical pain relief
- What kind of monitoring?
- Will I be allowed to eat?
- Episiotomy
- Acceleration
- Assisted delivery
- Caesarean options

There is little time to really promote the normality of birth and because the Dorothy in us wants everyone to feel good, we spend a lot of time promoting the normality of the *system.* Sarah works hard to ensure she uses inclusive and sensitive terminology such as referring to the major surgery of caesarean section as caesarean birth. But Paula wonders if this well-intentioned sensitivity helps, or instead, minimises the experience and contributes to normalising medical models of birth. She doubts whether the issues on the agenda previously referred to are the ones that really need addressing if the aim is to restore optimum levels of normality.

THE MISSING HISTORY OF CHILDBIRTH EDUCATION

It is interesting that as birth moved out of the home, so too did education for birth. The content of modern antenatal classes reflects the increased medicalisation of birth.

The providers of childbirth education are now specialists themselves – no longer simple sharers of wisdom, woman-to-woman, sister-to-sister (though secretly these networks are alive and well). And strangely, but not surprisingly, these educational specialists draw their authority from male teaching. Bradley, Lamaze, Dick-Read, Leboyer, Odent – it is these charismatic medical men we turn to for validation. But could this formalised and discrete approach to learning about birth be further undermining women's sense of their own innate knowledge and ability?

Wonderful and insightful as they were, these doctors did not pioneer childbirth education. Women have been sharing knowledge about birth with each other for millennia. Alongside strong oral routes of communication, there have been women who sought to educate a wider audience through the written word. I would like to introduce two women who made important contributions to childbirth education but are never celebrated in its history: Jane Sharp and Alice Bunker Stockham.

Jane Sharp published *The Midwives Book* in 1671 (edited by Hobby, 1999). She was the first 17th century British woman to publish such a text. It is thorough, learned and very accessible – indeed in the opening page of the fourth book she addresses herself to 'all women', as well as midwives, when she sets out the, 'rules for women that are come to their labour'. With her thirty years of experience, Jane understands much of what is considered good practice today. She cautions against unnecessary induction of labour, desiring, *all Midwives to take heed how they give anything inwardly to hasten the Birth, unless they are sure the Birth is at hand, many a child hath been lost for want of this knowledge* (p 159). She offers sensible pre-conceptual advice, describes perineal massage and herbal baths in pregnancy, and advises mobility in labour. Jane also recognises the importance of a wholesome diet and moderate exercise in ensuring a safe delivery, realising that *poor women are not able to provide in such cases, but their rich neighbours should do it for them; for I do not question but that all women will be glad to eat and drink well, and to take all things that may do them good if they knew but what, and can procure them* (p 141). To this end she provides a wealth of recipes for self-medication. Truly an empowering educational resource for women of her day – with much that is still current.

Alice Bunker Stockham, a friend of Leo Tolstoy, was the fifth woman to qualify as a doctor in the United States. She first published *Tokology – A Book for Every Woman*, in 1883. Apart from the remarkable wisdom and absolute truth that, 'No well regulated family should be without a hot water bottle' (Stockham 1907:115), Alice was a real pioneer of her times and has much to share with us even today. An advertisement for *Tokology,* in the back pages of the 1907 edition, reads:

> *Tokology teaches possible painless pregnancy and parturition, giving full, plain directions for the care of a woman before and after confinement. The ailments of pregnancy can be prevented as well as the pains and dangers of childbirth avoided WITHOUT DRUGS OR MEDICINES.*

At a time when it was illegal to do so, Alice ably and delicately addresses the issue of contraception. Exploring the commonly held belief that, *sexual union is a necessity to man, while it is not to woman* (p 152), Alice says of the young wife, *Neither has she learned that her body is her own and her soul is her Maker's. She gives up all ownership of herself to her husband, and what is the difference between her life and that of a public woman? She is sold to one man, and is not half so well paid* (pp 153-154).

Concerned with their economic plight, Alice had copies of *Tokology* privately printed and gave them to 'unfortunate women' to sell door-to-door in Chicago. Each copy came with a bound-in certificate signed by her, and entitling the bearer to a free gynaecological examination. A prime example of outreach work.

Alice recognises that the woman in labour, *is inclined to change [position] frequently, sitting, lying, walking and even kneeling* (p 177). She condemns *meddlesome midwifery* and says that *supporting the perineum is not only absolutely unnecessary, but also apt to be exceedingly injurious* (p 178). And she puts forward an interesting argument for not tying the umbilical cord. These are contemporary issues being openly discussed between women over a hundred years ago – a more comprehensive education for childbirth than we might see today.

What I noted with both these childbirth educators was their trust in a healthy woman's ability to cope with labour – they believed in her innate ability to give birth. The focus of their concern was on building health, in every sense, and providing the right environment and support for her during the birth.

The birth environment

Since we last met her, Kate has read a very interesting leaflet her midwife gave her and from this she has decided she would prefer not to have an epidural for pain relief except as an alternative to a general anaesthetic. She attends a course of excellent antenatal classes and learns about coping with normal labour in other ways. She feels strong, confident and excited in a way she hadn't thought possible before. If she succeeds in this she is going to enter parenthood feeling fantastic about herself, but if she finds for some reason she is unable to put this new learning into practice, she may feel very differently.

Identifying the factors that could empower or disempower Kate during her labour will enable Kate to pre-empt some potential problems and maximise her chances of a normal birth. This is one of the important roles of the childbirth educator.

We know that the same Kate, with the same background, will be much more likely to achieve her normal, epidural-free birth if she is in the right environment with the right people. Continuous emotional and physical support from another woman significantly shortens labour and decreases the need for caesarean deliveries, forceps and vacuum extraction, oxytocin augmentation and analgesia (Scott, Klaus, Klaus 1999).

Antenatal teachers can ask women to visualise their ideal birthing environment. Kate, like most women, envisages somewhere that does not remind her of operations – an environment that ensures her privacy, offers a range of places to be (being confined in one room is oppressive), and where she is free to labour in her own way, without routine procedures and time constraints. She pictures a midwife with a strong and genuine belief in the normality of birth, someone who is respectful and listens well, has time to give optimum care – in every sense – and is not disempowered by the system within which she works. While not entirely impossible, Kate will be lucky to realise this ideal by going into hospital.

Kate originally chose hospital birth to be 'on the safe side'. She felt that doctors have a lot of experience and wouldn't do anything to her that wasn't absolutely necessary.

For a healthy woman expecting a normal labour these premises are unsound. Should Kate's antenatal teacher disabuse her? Dorothy doesn't feel that it is her place to interfere – she is disempowered herself. Sarah is uncertain.

Disabuse is an interesting word. It means: to rid someone of a mistaken idea or impression. The word suggests that the act of allowing someone to remain under a false impression is abusive – a misuse of one's position or power. Sadly, some women do express feelings of having been manipulated, abused or traumatised during the course of their maternity care (Creedy, Shochet, Horsfall 2000; Kitzinger, 2001). Paula believes that good childbirth education is important because it can enable women to minimise this possibility and maximise the chances of having a positive birth experience. Women experience birth as positive if they feel in control of what happens to them (Johanson & Newburn, 2001) but birth plans are not always respected (Whitford & Hillan, 1998). Real empowerment might need to be achieved through the woman taking direct actions that shift the balance of power in her favour.

Figure 3.4
Women and health
professionals: The here and now
of immediacy of birth

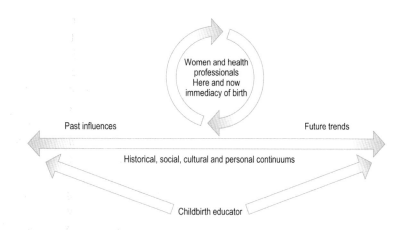

SHIFTING THE BALANCE OF POWER – THE IMPORTANCE OF THE CHILDBIRTH EDUCATOR

When I moved to rural Wales, my brother, concerned about my career, reminded me that sheep didn't need antenatal classes. This got me thinking – what if sheep flocked together and educated themselves – got wise? What if they developed assertiveness skills, took direct action, and decided not to lamb every year? Sheep farmers would feel pretty threatened by the prospect. Suppose for a moment that education for birth proved so effective that it threatened to bring about social change – a fifty per cent home birth rate for example. To facilitate this change there would need to be a shift in the current balance of power. People who hold power or authority now, would need to relinquish some. Having power, despite (or because of) the fact that it carries with it responsibility, makes us feel purposeful and important. And, as nobody is entirely altruistic, handing over power can feel diminishing and risky, and is therefore resisted. *Truly effective antenatal teachers must understand that they are likely to have their work sabotaged or disparaged in some way as part of this resistance.*

Childbirth educators are influential people. They can enable individuals to reclaim the power needed to make changes in their own lives and, through collective action, in society. Independent teachers are in a privileged position of not being disempowered by their place in a hierarchy. They are free to say what they see – and they are in a unique position to be able to take a wide view. Not being caught up in the day-to-day immediacy of maternity care in one particular setting, they can step back and examine the issues from wider and varied perspectives; and in doing so, contribute to our understanding about birth in an important way.

Medical and surgical skills play a vital part in the safe management of complicated pregnancies. However, where obstetricians have been allowed to define the parameters of normal birth, normal birth is in decline, with women feeling increasingly dissatisfied and disempowered by the experience.

While at present, childbirth education appears to be doing little to stem the rising tide of intervention, it *could* play a vital part in preserving the normality of birth and in enabling women to have an experience that is both enriching and empowering. Childbirth education is important when it strengthens women's belief in birth as a normal physiological process; it helps promote a cycle of belief and practice that supports the normality of birth, and it enables and supports women to make *and implement* decisions that will maximise their chances of the birth experience they hope for. Finally, and very importantly, education for birth can help build a community of birthing women by bringing together pregnant women with other women who have had positive and empowering experiences of birth in order for them to see that this is truly possible.

Figure 3.5
Learning and experience

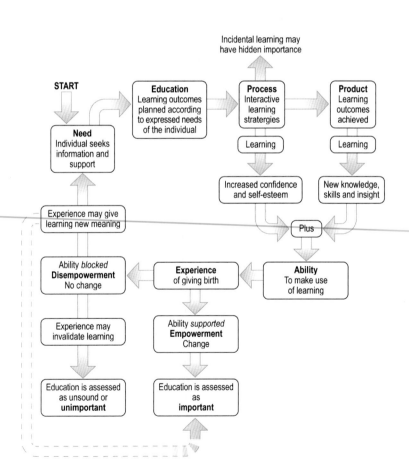

REFERENCES

Anderson T 2003 Antenatal classes: women-centred or service-driven? New Digest 22:11

Beech B 2000 Over-medicated and under-informed: what are the consequences for birthing women? Aims Journal 11(4):4-7

Berk L, Stanley T 1996 Therapeutic benefits of laughter. Online. Available: http://www.holistic-online.com/Humor_Therapy/humor_therapy_benefits.htm 7 May 2003

Bertin M Does the prenatal period influence our lives? Online Available:http://www.prenataleducation.org.uk/what_is_prenatal_education.htm 2 March 2003

Botella L Constructivism and narrative psychology. Online Available: http://www.infomed.es/constructivism/documsweb/andreas.html 1 April 2003

Chamberlain G, Wraight A, Crowley P (eds) 1997 Home births: the Report of the 1994 confidential enquiry by the National Birthday Trust fund. Parthenon Publishing Group, New York

Creedy D K, Shochet I M, Horsfall J 2000 Childbirth and the development of acute trauma symptoms: incidence and contributing factors. Birth 27(2):104-111

Henderson M 2002 Caesarean mothers risk losing chance to have more babies. Online. Available: http://www.timesonline.co.uk/article/0,,2-344309,00.html 7 May 2003

Hodnett E D 2002 The impact of childbirth experiences on women's sense of self: a review of the literature. Australian Journal of Midwifery 15(4):10-16

Johanson R, Newburn M 2001 Promoting normality in childbirth. British Medical Journal 323:1142-1143

Kirkham M, Stapleton H (eds) 2001 Executive summary: informed choice in maternity care: an evaluation of evidence based leaflets. NHS Centre for Reviews and Dissemination, York

Kitzinger S 2001 Becoming a mother. Midwifery Digest. 11:4

Leboyer F 1975 Birth without violence. Wildwood House, London

Manser M, Thomson M (eds) 1995 Chambers combined Dictionary Thesaurus. Chambers, Edinburgh

Miller J, Thornton E, Gittens C 2002 Influences of mode of birth and personality. British Journal of Midwifery 10 (11):692-697

National Childbirth Trust 2000 'Normal' birth is in decline. New Generation. Sept:7-11

Nichols F, Humenick S 2000 Childbirth education: practice, research and theory. W B Saunders, Philadelphia

Parliamentary Office of Science and Technology 2002 Postnote: caesarean sections. Online. Available: http://www.parliament.uk/post/home.htm 7 May 2003

Peterson G 1996 Childbirth: the ordinary miracle: effects of devaluation of childbirth on women's self-esteem and family relationships. Online. Available: http://www.birthpsychology.com/birthscene/mothers3.html 26 July 2003

Robertson A 1999 Empowering women. ACE Graphics, Australia

Scott K D, Klaus P H, Klaus M H 1999 The obstetrical and postpartum benefits of continuous support during childbirth. Journal of Women's Health Gender-based Medicine 8(10):1257-1264

Sharp J 1671 The midwives book: or the whole art of midwifery discovered. Hobby E (ed) 1999 Oxford University Press, Oxford

Simkin P 1992 Just another day in a woman's life? Part II: Nature and consistency of women's long-term memory of their first birth experiences. Birth 19(2):64-81

Stockham A 1907 Tokology: A book for every woman. Stockham, Chicago

Thomas J, Paranjothy S 2001 National sentinel caesarean section audit report. Royal College of Obstetricians and Gynaecologists Clinical Effectiveness Support Unit, RCOG Press, London

Vincent C, Neale G, Woloshynowych M 2001 Adverse events in British hospitals: preliminary retrospective record review. British Medical Journal 322:517-519

Waterstone M, Bewley S, Wolfe C 2001 Incidence and predictors of severe obstetric morbidity: case-control study. British Medical Journal 322:1089-1094

Whitford H, Hillan E 1998 Women's perceptions of birth plans. Midwifery 14(4):248-253

Young G, Hey E, Macfarlane A et al 2000 Choosing between home and hospital delivery. British Medical Journal 320:798

Chapter **4**

Birth and Parenting Education for Men

Adrienne Burgess and Tom Beardshaw

In recent years, there has been increased interest in the role of fathers in our society. Emerging from an era when many women chose to embark on motherhood without the support of a man, and when fathers were considered little more than a biological mechanism for the procreation of children, we have begun to realise that underfathered or unfathered children are disadvantaged compared with those who enjoy regular or even irregular fathering. The research now makes a strong case for involving men in early parenting. The need to provide education for men in the antenatal period would seem to be as urgent as it is for women. Little is currently known about what kind of antenatal education provision would best suit men, and what the content of sessions might be. However, there seems little doubt that these are issues which must now be addressed.

(Editors' note)

Today's new mothers and fathers face each other across a rapidly changing world. While mothers vary in their expectations about whether to 'do it all' or to stay in or out of the paid workforce and parent and toddler groups, they are often launched into motherhood without extended family support, due – among other things – to family networks that are smaller, weaker and more spread out geographically (Coffman et al, 1994). As for the fathers, although many work long hours, almost all want to 'do fatherhood' differently from previous generations, don't consider baby care un-masculine and think dads can be just as competent as mums (Lupton & Barclay, 1997). Cultural expectations and ideas abut gender roles are shifting. Across Europe, 86% of men (87% of women) now think fathers should be closely involved in child-rearing (Eurobarometer, 1992).

Many health professionals are responding to these new family circumstances and expectations. Weighing the assets available to the new mother and her baby, they have realised that one in particular is under-mobilised: the father. And also that when his contribution is minimal, this may not be due to unwillingness but can often be put down to institutional practices that do not help him develop sufficient skills and self-confidence (Lamb & Oppenheim, 1989).

> *In our new maternity unit in Grimsby a family is admitted to a single room for the whole duration of labour, delivery and postnatal care. Each room has en suite facilities and the woman's partner can stay overnight. In moving towards a new model of family centred care, fathers are brought into caring for their partners and infants. We expect this to free our midwives up to focus on the heart of their work; enable new fathers to be more effective at caring for their partners and babies; and improve the overall care that new mothers receive.*
>
> – Karen Robinson Head of Midwifery, Gynaecology & Sexual Health, North Lincolnshire and Goole Hospitals

Fathers are 'present' in the consciousness of perinatal workers as they have never been before, not only at the scans and births and antenatal sessions or in the line-up of media and sports stars showing caring and committed fathering as something to aspire to, but also, increasingly, in the home. When the health professional knocks on the door, it may be the father who opens it – thanks to his new right to paid paternity leave, or because he is working from home, is working shifts, or unemployed. And, especially if his partner is one of the 20% of mothers who has had a caesarean section and is not supposed to lift her baby, he may be holding that baby in his arms.

To health professionals, fathers can also be shadowy figures, as Bristol researcher Sue Pollock found while studying young fathers' experiences, when she noted that in 50% of cases health visitors did not even know their names – although the young mothers often placed a high value on their involvement (Pollock, 2001). Many such dads may have a tenuous connection with their 'baby mother', yet may want to be good fathers (Forrest, unpublished report, 2003).

> *The State of West Virginia found that the most significant person affecting whether a young man acknowledged he was the father was the midwife. The State implemented a training program for midwives on the importance of fatherhood and how to talk to young mothers and fathers. In four years the rate of 'paternity establishment' went from under 18% to over 60% among low-income unmarried couples.*
>
> – James Levine, Work and Families Institute, New York

The task of supporting men becoming fathers in the many types of families that populate Britain today is not simple. Families are culturally diverse; and there is no undisputed template of what a father should be. Nor can easy assumptions be made about fathers' expectations of health professionals. One may be keen to learn from a health visitor, and may even look to her for information about his own wellbeing; another may not look to her at all, construing contact with her as potentially 'offensive' (Williams, 1999). The aim of any family intervention is not to tell individuals, or communities, how to live their lives, but to harness their potential to find their own solutions. In working with expectant and new fathers, the aim does not need to be anything more complex than to include and encourage them.

But will this be of value? Can antenatal education in particular affect fathers' behaviour or experiences; mothers' behaviour or experiences; or child outcomes? Findings must be regarded with caution. Fathers who attend antenatal education may be unrepresentative; and programmes and outcome measures vary wildly. Evaluation of antenatal education for mothers faces similar problems, and robust findings in terms of benefits are hard to come by (for review, see Schmied et al, 1999). However, that does not mean initiatives are pointless or unfruitful. Lessons are being learned and small positive effects built on, to design new, and better, approaches.

> *Going skin-to-skin with new babies is a relatively new thing for fathers and not everybody approves. But it's only cuddling your baby, so why not? It's something dads want to do. And it's what they'll be doing if they're up half the night holding the baby. Men have totally changed in the course of my career. When I started out as a midwife 23 years ago, holding the baby in the delivery room was not where men were supposed to be. Now it's turned on its head. It's wonderful and skin-to-skin contact does help to bond fathers and children.*
>
> – Catherine Cummings, Senior Midwife, Forth Park Maternity Hospital, Fife

DADDY KNOW-NOTHING

Currently, few antenatal educators and programmes meet fathers' needs. McElligott (2001) found men keen to attend, but disappointed when they did. Smith (1999) found that during their partner's pregnancy men often feel in the 'back seat' and poorly informed. One man really valued a dads-only antenatal group because: 'It boosted my confidence when I talked to my wife. I has some ground to hold – I didn't feel completely ignorant' (Forrest, unpublished report, 2003).

Although it's now accepted that men can nurture, practice and much hard work are thought to be necessary for that nurturing capacity to emerge. Meanwhile, women are still assumed to 'know what to do' with babies and they are also encouraged to seek out information. There is a lot available to them, and their special worth as parents gets an extra boost from the current fashion for child-centred, empathy-based infant care, which values 'intuitive' (i.e. feminine) response and immediate gratification of babies' needs (Lupton & Barclay, 1997).

Fathers are keen to learn from their partners, and feel they need new practical and emotional skills to achieve their goal of 'doing fatherhood' differently (Lupton & Barclay, 1997). However, they rarely study 'pregnancy' literature. Many try and then discard it, finding it condescends to them or is mother-focused (Lewis, 1986). Until genuinely father-directed perinatal literature is widely available, this avenue of learning is likely to be closed to many expectant fathers. Videos/DVDs may appeal, and may not be so mother-directed. And antenatal educators can refer fathers to websites where they can obtain information and chat to other dads (e.g. www.fathersdirect.com – expectant and new dads are among its heaviest users).

Antenatal education: what dads want (taken from Forrest, 2003)

- A male facilitator - who is a father himself
- Someone to answer obstetric questions
- To hear from dads who are already dads (videos of new dads talking; a 'real' dad visiting the group, hopefully with his baby)
- Information: 'I was hungry for information - I didn't know what I needed to know'.
- Challenge: 'I was worried about being at the birth ... he (the facilitator) really challenged me'
- Accreditation: 'I am going to court. It would help me to show I had done this course'.
- Handouts: 'It feels like there is so much more to find out'
- To pay: 'You could charge - it would ensure commitment and firm up the group'

Since successful fatherhood is portrayed as something essentially learned, men may welcome formal birth and parenting 'training' ('education' or 'support' may not be terms that appeal to them), especially if it is offered at a time most could attend (e.g. evening/Saturday mornings), as a routine intervention (rather than one for 'problem' dads) and as a continuing part of a pre-birth programme. One study found 4 out of 5 fathers of six-month-olds saying they would probably have attended a 'how to care for your baby' session, if it had been offered in the first few weeks after the birth and as a continuation of their pre-birth training. Although when new fathers were actually offered such a session only 1 in 6 attended, the researchers felt this was a very positive result, since in that district nothing of that kind had ever been offered before (Matthey & Barnett, 1999).

In England and Wales, a health visitor intervention at six weeks post partum may eventually be routine (Henricson, 2003). Since this is the peak time for babies' crying, and for babies being shaken, work with fathers as well as mothers might be particularly valuable at this point. Given fathers' low-level knowledge base, programmes must include information on infant development, so that fathers can be helped to develop realistic expectations of their baby's needs and capabilities.

A prenatal US project with low-income fathers provided each man with two one-and-a-half hour sessions of factual information and practical skills training. Fathers were also informed of the unborn's unique personality and capacity to hear and respond to a familiar voice; and attempts were made to induce intrauterine bonding of father to unborn baby (which a number of studies have shown as proving successful in prenatal childbirth classes). One month postnatally the men were videoed with their babies, and their knowledge of infant cues and development tested. The information had been retained to a remarkable degree, and the 'intervention' group scored much more highly than a comparison group.

– Pfannenstiel & Honig (1995)

Supporting fathers during pregnancy

It's worth noting that expectant fathers who receive emotional support have better physical and emotional health (Jones, 1988, cited by Diemer, 1997), which very probably translates into being 'easier to live with', and more supportive and positive. But emotional support may not be something expectant fathers easily come by: most normally seek this from their partner, but hesitate to do so when she is pregnant, leaving themselves emotionally isolated when numerous new concerns and worries are entering their lives (Lewis, 1986). Group- and discussion-based antenatal education may provide opportunities for such support, or may help the expectant father to see when he can, in fact, seek this from his partner.

Fathers' key concerns relating to the pregnancy include: 'something being wrong with the baby'; 'what if there's a miscarriage'; and 'what can I do to help my partner through pregnancy' (Lupton & Barclay, 1997). Other worries include feeling 'not ready' to be a father, which may include the timing of the pregnancy, the quality of the couple's relationship, and money worries (Jackson, 1986). Men who are obstructive or attention-seeking during sessions may be signalling distress. Antenatal education cannot meet all clients' needs, so referral systems need to be in place to cope with, among other things, substance abuse, domestic violence, debt problems, and serious couple issues. However, impending fatherhood should not be pathologised: most expectant fathers are tremendously happy and excited, and this should be acknowledged.

There is evidence that even traditional antenatal education can reduce some fathers' fears and anxieties. Maybe partly because of this,

Topics of interest to fathers (McElligott, 2001)

- The father's role
- Care of the baby after delivery
- What could go wrong
- Physical and emotional changes
- Stages of labour
- When to seek help
- Pain relief in labour
- Premature delivery
- Postnatal depression

antenatal attendance by the couple often leads to greater mutual dependence and more supportive behaviours (for review, see Diemer, 1997). Diemer found fathers who attend antenatal sessions are more likely to turn to other people as a means of coping (i.e. to use 'social support'); and also to do more housework (a very practical way of providing support) than fathers who don't attend. When antenatal sessions are specifically designed to identify and meet fathers' own needs and concerns, the impact can be even more positive, with the attending men using even more 'social support', doing even more housework, being more likely to 'reason' with their partners, and reporting better overall relationships with them (Diemer, 1997).

Fathers may not always need to 'talk about' things to feel better: we came across a local NCT fathers' group that had been set up by a man whose partner had suffered from postnatal depression. Other men in the same situation had joined, and the group had been very supportive. Formal discussion, however, did not figure in their meetings: the men played five-a-side football, and then 'had a pint'. Since regular exercise is a known mood-lightener (and can even help in the alleviation of clinical depression) this might not be a bad strategy.

Preparing fathers for the birth

Even when expectant fathers haven't had any training, most mothers want them present at the birth, and find it beneficial. Since almost all fathers are now present, the benefits can be hard to measure as there is no comparable 'control group' of non-attending fathers for viable

Topics of relatively little interest to fathers (McElligott, 2001)

- Bottle feeding technique
- Discomforts of pregnancy
- Benefits of breastfeeding
- Positions for delivery[1]

---

[1]Fathers also expressed little interest in 'family dynamics' but since they had evinced substantial interest in learning about other 'emotional' topics, McElligott concluded that they hadn't understood the term!

comparison. However, a body of research has shown that mothers whose partners are with them during labour and delivery are less distressed, experience less pain, receive less medication and feel more positive about the birth experience (for review see Lamb, 1997; also Tarkka, 2000). Mothers rate the father's presence as significantly more helpful than that of nurses; and while mothers are generally disappointed by the level of midwife involvement, their partner's involvement much more nearly meets their expectations (Spiby et al, 1999). Obstetricians greatly underestimate the psychological boost fathers give to their partners during delivery – as well as the practical support they provide during labour, and afterwards: their contribution as a general factotum on understaffed labour wards cannot be overestimated (Hayward & Chalmers, 1990).

We want the father to be part of the experience. We find him invaluable. It is very different when the woman does not have him there. The midwives have to do far more. The father is vital, particularly if she has had a caesarean or stitches. He is always busy, running baths, getting drinks, helping her to the bathroom, lifting the baby, sharing the responsibility. She has her own helper – the person who cares about her more than anyone else in the world.

– Caroline Flint, ex-President of the Royal College of Midwives and Founder of the Tooting Birth Centre, London

Today, much antenatal labour-preparation for fathers is minimal. Even so, it can be positive. Prepared fathers tend to be more active participants, and their partners' birth experiences better (for review, see Diemer, 1997). Really well-prepared fathers might contribute much more, since when labour partners know a lot about pain control, women have shorter labours and are less likely to have epidurals (studies cited by Enkin et al, 1995). It has been noted that fathers tend to play different roles during labour – e.g. as 'coach, partner or bystander' (Chapman, 1991, cited by Larimore, 1999). To our knowledge, no thorough trainings have been developed to discuss such choices for fathers. In fact, we have not seen even a really good list of the things fathers can 'do' during labour. Many would find such a list invaluable (Lupton & Barclay, 1997). Some practitioners have commented that to expect a father to act as a 'coach' runs the risk of setting him up for failure. That, and other related issues, merit examination and discussion.

Men-only and women-only sessions as a component of antenatal education are generally welcomed by both men and women, with most men reporting they feel more confident and better prepared if they can discuss issues with other fathers-to-be. An expectant father is more inclined to attend an antenatal course if it has been recommended by a male personal contact (McElligott, 2001) and every project that has trialled these has found them highly valued by the fathers. Where the entire antenatal programme is built on couple participation, women too have valued the single-sex groups.

> *A pilot scheme in Australia suggested both mothers and fathers appreciate it if the antenatal class is split part of the time, so we tried it at the Dundee & Perth Royal Infirmary. For seven months, a male facilitator was there to lead discussion among dads at two of the three evening classes. Men liked having something just for them and they asked questions ranging from 'how do you hold a baby' to 'how is this going to change my life?' The men ended up being more aware and better informed than they might have been otherwise. If only we could do this all the time – but it costs money and properly qualified male facilitators are hard to find.*

– Dr Andrew Symon, Dundee University

Fathers worry about how their partner will manage the pain of the birth (Lupton & Barclay, 1997). Demonstrating the passage of the baby using a life size pelvis and doll to confirm the perfect fit of mother and baby has been found useful (Steiner Celebi, 2003). Presenting a clear and realistic picture of the available pain relief and possible medical interventions is clearly necessary, but educators are advised not to launch into a lecture, before finding out how much the group already knows. A need to 'plug gaps' may emerge.

One practitioner believes it is crucial to explain, cognitively, the importance of relaxation and how this relates to the release of endorphins and oxytocin, since this provides the rationale for fathers to learn massage skills and so on (Steiner Celebi, 2003). Together, the men and their partners can identify and repeatedly practise relaxation /coping strategies, such as sighing-out-slowly and Laura Mitchell relaxation and postural change; and identify other strategies, such as particular music, visualisations and shared memories. Women must also be helped to communicate when these are not working. Both partners can practise these as relaxation strategies for any stressful situation, not only for labour. This wider application may be useful to both partners, and 'doing' rather than just watching or coaching may help the expectant father truly understand the technique, and be able to help his partner practise more effectively at home. It is hypothesised that one of the reasons many women do not properly use, during labour, techniques learned in class, is that they have not practised them enough.

Fathers can be empowered to question medical interventions and negotiate with health professionals: a technique such as BRAIN (what are the Benefits, Risks, Alternatives, Intuition and likely outcomes of doing Nothing) could help with decision making during labour, as well as providing a rationale to help the man support his partner at home or stay with her in hospital in pre-labour, when many are encouraged to leave.

Fathers should also be encouraged to think about the kind of support they themselves will need, if they are to support their partners effectively during labour and delivery. And to recognise that theirs is not purely a support role: they are also there in their own right – as the father of the child (Lee & Schmied, 2001).

> **Father-friendly practice in labour and delivery** (Adapted from Lee & Schmied, 2001)
>
> - Make the couple aware that they are free to choose whether the father attends the birth or not, and that there is a range of roles he can play during labour.
> - Find out from him and the mother what kind of role(s) they would like him to play.
> - Let the father-to-be know that his presence can be very reassuring - he can be useful just by being there.
> - Learn his name, make eye contact and smile at him!
> - Where appropriate, make suggestions to him about how he can offer practical help - perhaps with small tasks, massage, lifting or touch.
> - Keep him involved in conversations about the progress of labour and, if appropriate, about decisions on interventions and pain relief.
> - If his partner is taken into surgery, make sure he is OK.

Involving new fathers at home

Why should perinatal education support fathers' involvement at home? Fathers are the closest source of emotional support available to most new mothers (Levitt et al, 1995, cited by Baafi et al, 2001); and though mothers' support groups are valued, the evidence is that this is no substitute for a caring and supportive father (Cowan, 1988; Lieberman, 1981). When fathers are strongly supportive and helpful, mothers are less likely to suffer from postnatal depression (Levitt, 1993); and tend to be more closely bonded to their children, more responsive and more sensitive to their needs (Fearing, cited in Lamb, 1997). Since new mothers commonly feel overburdened and 'who is doing (or not doing) what' is a common source of discord and stress for couples (Barclay & Lupton, 1999), supporting effective father-involvement postnatally has to be important and useful.

The babies benefit, too: those who experience positive, high-level engagement with their fathers in the first four weeks of life are performing better than their peers on their first birthdays; and well-fathered six and seven year olds not only achieve better at school (socially and academically) but register higher IQs (Pleck, 1997). There is also a strong correlation between father involvement at 18 months and six years; and between father involvement at age 7 and the number of national examination passes at age 16; as well as the likelihood of having a criminal record by age 21 – the higher the father involvement, the less likely a criminal record (studies cited by Lewis, 2001). This kind of finding holds, whether fathers are living with their children or not (Amato & Gilbreth, 1999).

How well do ordinary antenatal sessions prepare fathers to be usefully participative at home? Not well. Singh and Newburn (2000) found one man in three wanting more information on a range of nineteen subjects. Fathers are concerned that they lack the skills or confidence to look after a baby, or adopt a proper fatherly role. They want information on what to expect of life with a new baby, practical tips on baby care, and advice on being part of a new family (for review, see Fathers Direct, 2001).

We always ask new mums how they felt about their visit to the hospital, and use the information to develop and improve our service. We have recently extended this and now we give the new dads a questionnaire as well. This is helping us to understand their feelings and needs and make small changes to the maternity unit that improve things for the father. We have special visiting hours for partners – they are treated differently from normal 'visitors' so that they can be with their partner and baby for much longer than would have been the case. We also make sure that education about important information and skills – such as bathing the baby – is done when the fathers are there as well, and not when the mothers are there alone.

– Diane Paterson, Development Manager, Queen Mother Hospital, Glasgow

Do fathers have to be extensively trained if they are to take more responsibility for infant care? Not necessarily. The simple opportunity to undertake parenting in a supportive environment can increase their caretaking. Keller (1985, cited by Lamb, 1997) found that fathers who were extensively engaged with their new babies in the hospital setting tended to stay closely involved when their infant came home. And Palkovitz (1982) found that enabling a new father to spend a lot of time at the hospital, and facilitating early (and extended) father–infant contact, were associated with relatively high levels of paternal caregiving and social involvement when the baby was five months old. Lewis (1986) noted that fathers could feel inhibited if experienced mothers were watching them, so creating a private space for them to 'practise' (for example, drawing curtains round the bed) may be helpful. Fathers' greatest fears in terms of handling newborns are that they will look clumsy and stupid, and that their 'big hands' or lack of manual dexterity will harm the infant (Lewis, 1986; Lupton & Barclay, 1997). Fathers are also very open to talking about their hopes and fears during this time; and Anderson (1996) suggests that midwives help them explore these, as well as including them in infant care.

Why can the simple opportunity to get some practice in, deliver such benefits? Probably because very few fathers get much chance to practise. Yet practice seems to be one of the most important things, if fathers are to be actively involved. There is a 'virtuous circle' here: a sense of 'mastery' (being able to change a baby efficiently or settle it effectively) can deliver satisfaction. And the more a father does, the more confident and relaxed his approach is, and the more familiar he feels to the baby – who is then more likely to respond positively to his handling. This positive response further encourages the father, who then does more caretaking – and the circle continues. For fathers, 'need' often provides opportunity: fathers of caesarean or premature babies tend to be more involved than many other fathers, and often develop the same skills as mothers in caring for them (Parke, 1981).

Fathers' skills and self-confidence are vulnerable. An intrusive 'coach', be they the mother or a health professional, who makes disapproving faces or re-does something he has just done, can cause him to withdraw. Skill difference between themselves and their partner also seems to be an inhibitor; and if fathers who have been very involved get 'out of practice', they can withdraw again (Lupton & Barclay, 1997). Simply explaining these processes to parents (mothers as well as fathers) may be useful. And it may also be useful to explain that a parent doesn't have to be eyeball to eyeball with their infant 24 hours per day to develop sufficient 'sensitivity'. An Israeli study found that when employed fathers of nine-month-olds spent as little as 45

Recommendations for father-friendly practice (adapted from Singh & Newburn, 2000)

- Identify local fathers: their names, addresses and relationship to child and mother
- Identify the information and support needs of these men
- Develop and publish an information and support strategy for fathers
- Develop niche- and direct-marketing to fathers, and to different groups of fathers (e.g. low income or ethnic minority fathers)
- Include pictures of fathers in posters and handouts
- Collect and provide other resources 'for dads'
- Train and support staff to engage positively with men, in styles they find useful and acceptable
- Train and support staff to deliver information and skills training to fathers
- Consider ways of keeping fathers 'in the picture', for example reviewing visiting hours, timing of antenatal sessions, flexible out-of-hours work by health professionals, and/or making it possible for fathers to stay overnight after the birth

minutes per day actively engaged with them, they 'knew' them as well as the non-employed mothers: in interaction, they were no less likely to offer the appropriate toy or response, which in turn stimulated the baby to an active and positive response (Ninio & Rinott, 1988).

Actually training the fathers up in infant care (i.e. doing more than simply giving them the opportunity to do it) can deliver even greater participation. In Sweden, Lind (1974, cited by Lamb, 1997) found that fathers who were taught how to care for their newborns, and were encouraged to do so, were more involved three months later. Similarly McHale et al (1984, cited by Lamb, 1997) found that fathers who thought of themselves as more skilled were more involved. None of this is surprising, since willingness to undertake a task – any task – is often strongly linked with confidence; and confidence is strongly linked with skills.

Men's learning skills in caring for the infant appeared to be a crucial step in their becoming closer to the child. Even those fathers who saw their participation as limited ... started to feel satisfaction ... when they felt they had 'succeeded' in a task ... Those men who did not enter into close, care-providing relationships in the early weeks and months of their child's life took longer to gain rewards from their children.

– Lupton & Barclay (1997)

WHAT ARE FATHERS FOR?

Most expectant and new fathers put 'the father's role' as their top concern. Breadwinning is a major issue. Many couples regard this as the father's responsibility in an emotional and ideological sense, even if the mother is the main wage earner; and men who feel they are failing in the breadwinner role can withdraw for that reason (Warin et al, 1999). Women whose partners suggest that they might perhaps be the one to 'stay home' may knock the idea back without further discussion, or without considering other alternatives (Lupton & Barclay, 1997).

Where substantial paid work is not an option, fathers may need to be helped to see other important roles for themselves. In fact, many mothers take on a breadwinning role; and today's couples make diverse and complex choices about division of responsibilities, often based on very simple financial maths. 'Going back to work' is usually presented in perinatal education as a 'woman's choice' (e.g. Ockenden, 1998). Men are assumed to have no 'right' to choose. Father-inclusive practice would shift the paradigm away from 'mother's choice' to family choice about creating a mix of work and childcare that connects the needs of the child to the aspirations of both new mother and father. While it is often said that new fathers work particularly long hours, recent samples reveal a mixed picture: Baafi et al (2001) found 60% of new fathers maintaining their usual working hours; 12% working more hours (often in second jobs, to make up for their partner's absence from the labour market); and 28% working fewer hours.

With discussion centred on work–life balance for both partners, other issues may emerge. Both mothers and fathers increasingly express dissatisfaction with their own and their partner's role performance (Lupton & Barclay, 1997). Once, 'traditional' couples had the highest post-birth satisfaction. Today, while some of these still manage the transition to parenthood well, post-birth satisfaction for both partners is increasingly linked to role-flexibility (Lupton & Barclay, 1997). While most new fathers are disappointed by the relatively small baby involvement their work allows them, many do not know how to advocate for themselves in the workplace, or how to 'work smarter'. Unconscious beliefs – regarding, for example, the unacceptability of letting workmates down – can also hamper discussion. Father-inclusive antenatal practice would include information about paternity leave and other statutory rights, such as the right to ask for flexible working. Some fathers will need information about child support and Parental Responsibility law.

Parents speaking of the impact on their parenting practices of a non-traditional antenatal class in Coff's Harbour, New South Wales, Australia:

FATHER: The class made me very conscious of how important it is to be involved from the start.

MOTHER: It was really important that I was educated that dads help out.

(Russell, unpublished paper, 2003)

Identifying fathers' concerns, and thinking them through, can help educators tackle areas in which fathers have traditionally shown little interest. For example, fathers, like mothers, are keen to acquire confidence and skills to use the health care system effectively and make decisions about their families' health and care (Nolan, 1999). Setting discussions such as breast and bottle feeding, smoking, diet, exercise and so on within that context, may be a way forward.

An issue emerging as problematic from perinatal research is that of 'father as playmate'. Many Western fathers see shared recreational activities with their child (often in a sporting context) as the primary means of developing a close and loving relationship with them. So when confronted with a tiny and not obviously 'social' infant, many new fathers draw back, unable to work out how to 'play' with such a tiny child or to see another role for themselves (Lupton & Barclay, 1997).

Parents offered traditional perinatal care in Coff's Harbour, NSW

FATHER: There was nothing for the fathers really. I eavesdropped so I guess I learned a bit.

MOTHER: The nurse ... asked why the father should bath the baby ... [she said] that men make life more complicated and he should come back later. (Russell, unpublished paper, 2003)

Matthey and Barnett (1999) believe fathers would respond well to the Brazleton method of infant assessment/stimulation, which could show them age-appropriate techniques for 'play', and reveal their newborn's capacities for reciprocal communication. Fathers might also be helped to broaden the notion of 'play', for example to understand that for babies 'play' and 'care' can be indistinguishable: much play happens during nappy changes, feeding, bathing and so on. The value of participating in such activities can also be promoted to the many new fathers who cannot see a role for themselves when their babies are breastfed, and who often withdraw in disappointment (Lupton & Barclay, 1997). Later, other care activities (such as cooking for and with a child, shopping together, choosing clothes to wear in the morning) can also be revealed as the kinds of shared activities likely to foster the loving closeness that almost all fathers look for.

Another role fathers anticipate and think about, is that of protector/disciplinarian (Lupton & Barclay, 1997). Fathers, more than mothers, look at their newborns and worry about schooling, drugs, the 'right' behaviour for a father (do I have to be strict?). This concern can provide antenatal educators with a starting point for discussion about productive and age-appropriate parenting styles. Making fathers aware of other parenting courses, and facilitating connections with them, may build a valuable continuum of education and support. A London father from an antenatal dads' group went on to a Positive Parenting course (Forrest, unpublished report, 2003).

> Now I am going to Positive Parenting class, I am the only guy with ten women, I am proud of this too. Our health visitor recommended it. I love it. It's just local women and me and we maybe watch a video and then talk about it.
>
> – London father interviewed by Forrest, Working with Men Evaluation, unpublished report

A FINAL WORD

Since mothers are currently fathers' main source of education and support (Lupton & Barclay, 1997) equipping mothers with information for fathers and explaining how to support them can be of value. One significant finding is that men who feel supported by their partners in finding their own ways of doing things are likely to develop a strong connection to their infants, and are unlikely to develop depression (Cowan, 1988). Lupton and Barclay (1997) found that the mothers who were most insistent about the 'rightness' of taking on full responsibility for infant care themselves were not necessarily those most suited to the job; sometimes they clung on out of desperation, and fear of failure. Mothers may also want contradictory things (Jordan, 1995, cited by Lupton & Barclay, 1997): to take control of their partner's activities in childcare and position themselves as primary parent, yet to have him 'help'. It is not always easy to recognise such complexities. Nor is it always easy to 'see' what a father wants. The 'deficit perspective' on fathers is widespread (Hawkins & Dollahite, 1997), expressing itself in such beliefs as those shown in the box below.

The defecit perspective on fathers

- 'A father cannot cope with children without a woman to help him.'
- 'A father is not interested in the caring role unless there is a woman who is pushing him.'
- 'A man is unwilling to change.'
- 'An absent father has little influence on a child's development.'
- 'An absent father who has no relationship with the child is avoiding his responsibilities and needs to be punished.'
- 'Men are not particularly motivated by their status as a parent. Their main interest is a job.'
- 'Men are worse at 'multi-tasking' and less cooperative and so they are less good at parenting and they cannot learn.'
- 'Men are in crisis.'
- 'Men who are concerned about these issues have a secret 'men's rights' agenda, rather than a genuine interest in the needs of children.'
- 'A teenage father is not interested in the child and avoids his responsibilities.'
- 'Men are intrinsically violent and this is not treatable.'
- 'Men are much more likely to harm a child than women.'
- 'Men's role as protectors of children at risk of abuse is limited.'
- 'A man showing concerns for a child other than his own in a public place is likely to be a paedophile.'
- 'Domestic violence is perpetrated by men (only) on women (only). One in four fathers beats their partner.'

Where these beliefs are held by the father or his partner or powerful health professionals, his interest in playing a significant part in infant care may not be seen at all. A more fruitful approach is to assume that a new father is interested in learning how to care for his baby, and to work to build his confidence and competence. Infant care can be presented as an opportunity to hone skills he is no less capable than his partner of acquiring; and he will be intrigued to learn that research has shown men to be no less sensitive to babies' cries than women, and that, given the same opportunities, education and support, that men learn child-care skills at exactly the same rate as women (Lewis, 2001).

A final few thoughts on father–friendly practice

- For managers: identify any barriers to engaging fathers and seek to resolve them.
- Make fathers feel welcome at all times
- Wherever appropriate (i.e. according to the woman's wishes) encourage men to be actively involved in the decision making process regarding their baby.
- Include fathers in any teaching about caring for the baby.
- Help men to decide what they need to know.
- Give fathers an opportunity to discuss their thoughts and feelings about the birth and the baby and becoming a parent - with their partners present, and perhaps also separately
- Consider using male facilitators and some men-only discussion groups - splitting the couples up also gives women some 'women only' time.
- Try to avoid the word 'parent': it will usually be heard as 'mother'. If a service is for mums only say so; if it's for both parents, say mums and dads.

BIBLIOGRAPHY AND REFERENCES

Amato P R, Gilbreth J C G 1999 Non-resident fathers and children's wellbeing: a meta-analysis. Journal of Marriage and the Family 55:23-38

Anderson A M 1996 The father – infant relationship: becoming connected. Journal of Social and Paediatric Nursing 1(2):83-92

Baafi M, McVeigh C, Williamson M 2001 Fatherhood: the changes and the challenges. British Journal of Midwifery 9(9):567-570

Barclay L, Lupton D 1999 The experiences of new fatherhood: a socio-cultural analysis. Journal of Advanced Nursing 29(4):1013-1020

Burghes L, Clarke L, Cronin N 1997 Fathers and fatherhood in Britain. FPSC, London

Burgess A 1996 Fatherhood reclaimed: the making of the modern father. Vermilion, London

Coffman S, Levitt M, Brown L 1994 Effects of clarification of support expectations in prenatal couples. Nursing Research 43:111-116

Cowan C P 1988 Working with men becoming fathers: the impact of a couples group intervention. In: Bronstein P, Cowan C P (eds) The transition to parenthood: how a first child changes a marriage. John Wiley, New York

Davidson N, Lloyd T 1995 Working with men. Teenage Parenthood Network June:10-12

Diemer G A 1997 Expectant fathers: influence of perinatal education on stress, coping and spousal relations. Research in Nursing and Health 20:281-293

Enkin M W, Keirse M J N C, Neilson J et al 1995 A guide to effective care in pregnancy and childbirth. Oxford University Press, Oxford

Eurobarometer 1993 Europeans and the family. European Commission, Brussels

Fathers Direct 2001 How to build new dads. Factsheet. Online. Available: http://www.fathersdirect.com

Hawkins A J, Dollahite D C (eds) 1997 Generative fathering: beyond deficit perspectives. Sage, Thousand Oaks, CA

Hayward J, Chalmers B 1990 Obstetricians' and mothers' perceptions of obstetric events. Journal of Psychosomatic Obstetrics and Gynaecology 11(1)

Henneborn W J, Cogan R 1975 The effect of husband participation on reported pain and probability of medication during labor and birth. Journal of Psychosomatic Research 19(3):215-222

Henricson C 2003 Government and parenting. Joseph Rowntree Foundation, York

Jackson B 1986 Fatherhood. Allen & Unwin, London

Kocher N 1987 West Germany and the German-speaking countries. In: Lamb M E (ed) The father's role: cross cultural perspectives. Lawrence Erlbaum, Hillsdale, New Jersey

Lamb M E, Oppenheim D 1989 Fatherhood and father – child relationships: five years of research. In: Cath S H, Gurwitt A, Gunsberg L (eds) Fathers and their families. Analytic Press, Hillsdale, New Jersey

Lamb M E 1997 The development of father – infant relationships. In: Lamb M E (ed) The role of the father in child development, 3rd edn. John Wiley, New York

Larimore W L 1999 The role of the father in childbirth. Midwifery Today 51: 15-17

Lee J, Schmied V 2001 Involving men in antenatal education. British Journal of Midwifery 9(9):559-561

Levitt M J 1993 Social support and relationship change after childbirth: an expectancy model. Health Care Women International 14:503-512

Lewis C 1986 Becoming a father. Open University Press, Milton Keynes

Lewis C 2001 What good are dads? Factsheet by Fathers Direct, NFPI, NEWPIN. Working with men, London

Lieberman M A 1981 The effects of social support on responses to stress. Free Press, New York

Lupton D, Barclay L 1997 Constructing fatherhood: discourses and experiences. Sage, London

Matthey S, Barnett B 1999 Parent– infant classes in the early postpartum period: need and participation by fathers and mothers. Infant Mental Health Journal 20(3):278-290

McElligott M 2001 Antenatal information wanted by first-time fathers. British Journal of Midwifery 9(9):556-558

Meighan M, Davis M W, Thomas S P et al 1999 Living with postpartum depression: the father's experience. American Journal of Maternal/Child Nursing 24(4):202-209

Ninio A, Rinott N 1988 Fathers' involvement in the care of their infants and their attributions of cognitive competence to infants. Child Development 59:652-663

Nolan M L 1999 Antenatal education: past and future agendas. Practising Midwife 2(3):24-27

Ockenden J 1998 Antenatal education for parenting. In: Nolan M L (ed) Education and support for parenting. Baillière Tindall, London

Palkovitz R 1982 Fathers' birth attendance, early extended contact, and father– infant interaction at five months postpartum. Birth 9(3):173-177

Parke R D 1981 Fathering. Collins, London

Pfannenstiel A E, Honig A S 1995 Effects of a prenatal 'Information and insights about infants' program on the knowledge base of first-time low-education fathers one month postnatally. Early Child Development and Care 111:87-105

Pleck J H 1997 Paternal involvement: levels, sources and consequences In: Lamb M E (ed) The role of the father in child development, 3rd edn. John Wiley, New York

Pollock S 2001 Focus: Young fathers. Young People's Health Network. Health Development Agency 15

Schmied V, Myors K, Wills J 1999 'Visions' of parenthood: innovation in the presentation of childbirth and parenting education. Family Health Research Unit, St. George's Hospital, Sydney

Schott J, Priest J 2002 Leading antenatal classes, 2nd edn. Butterworth Heinemann, Oxford

Singh D, Newburn M 2000 Becoming a father: men's access to information and support about pregnancy, birth and life with a new baby. National Childbirth Trust and Fathers Direct, London

Smith N 1999 Antenatal classes and the transition to fatherhood: a study of some fathers' views. MIDIRS Midwifery Digest 9(4): 463-468

Spiby H, Henderson B, Slade P et al 1999 Strategies for coping with labour: does antenatal education translate into practice? Journal of Advanced Nursing 29(2):388

Steiner Celebi M 2003 Preparing for the birth. Online. fathers. moni@ymte.co.uk

Tarkka M T, Paunonen M, Laippala P 2000 Importance of the midwife in the first-time mother's experience of childbirth. Scandinavian Journal of Caring Sciences 14:3:184-190

Warin J, Solomon Y, Lewis C et al 1999 Fathers, work and family life. Joseph Rowntree Foundation, York

Williams R 1999 Going the distance: fathers, health and health visiting. Dept. of Professional Education in Community Studies, Reading

Chapter **5**

Are Midwives Empowered Enough to Offer Empowering Education?

Sara Wickham and Lorna Davies

In the UK, midwives provide the vast majority of antenatal and early postnatal education for women and their families. It has been suggested that the position of midwives and midwifery skills – increasingly subservient to medical staff and to a medical/risk-orientated philosophy of birth – makes it difficult for midwives to offer empowering antenatal education which embodies respect for the adulthood of expectant parents. When staff are not themselves respected for their skills, do not feel strong within the system of maternity care, and are bound by hospital policies and protocols, it may be hard for them to educate women about their choices and to foster confidence in their inner resources. Educating midwives to be change agents in the maternity care services may need to precede their engaging in practice as childbirth educators.

(Editors' note)

It might seem a bit passé to begin this chapter by referring to the distinction between teaching for compliance, teaching for persuasion and teaching for change (Priest & Schott, 1994), yet this is the crux of the issue we are debating in this book. As women and midwives who feel empowered ourselves, one of our goals is in doing whatever we can to enable other women to hold their own power – whether this relates to the decisions that they make, or simply to the way they feel about themselves as women. As midwife educators who regularly assess antenatal education sessions offered by student and qualified midwives, we see a wide range; from those which effectively teach women to be 'good girls' and behave within the system, quashing all notion of choice, to those which are truly emancipatory, offering tools for liberation. The majority of the sessions that we see sit somewhere between these two extremes.

The concept of empowerment is complex, multidimensional and laden with a range of meanings (Too, 1996). Some authors have found it easier to define the absence of empowerment, using terms such as learned helplessness, powerlessness, dependency and victimisation (Rappaport, 1984; Wallerstein, 1992; Too, 1996), while Merali (2001) proposes a more positively-focused definition: that being empowered is about having control over one's destiny. Flint (1990) once pointed out that the moment a woman becomes a mother is the point at which she needs to feel at her most powerful, in order to fulfil this role to the best of her ability. Yet Davis-Floyd (1992) shows that the rituals which have developed around birth in modern Western culture effectively socialise women into being passive 'patients', who may then teach the same passivity and conformity to their own children. As a consequence, many women leave their experience of the maternity services feeling disempowered, and with their needs unmet.

Our own view on the definition of empowerment is that it is not as simple as coming up with a prescription which helps empower somebody else, although until fairly recently some people talked and wrote as if it was. In the same way that you can take the proverbial horse to water but not be able to control whether or not it drinks, the choice to become empowered is something that needs to come from within. In theory, it is possible – and potentially desirable – to offer experiences and tools which enable the person to see what empowerment looks like, and how it might be achieved. In our experience of working to enable the empowerment of midwives and childbearing women there seems to be something as yet intangible which is the key ingredient in women 'finding themselves'.

In some ways, it is difficult to separate out the contact that midwives have with women during antenatal education sessions from the contact they have with women throughout the whole childbirth experience. Although scheduled sessions may comprise the main opportunity that most women and their partners have to think about their choices and plans, in an ideal world midwives will continually offer women education in an empowering way, in order to help them to grow through the journey of childbirth. This chapter, then, will explore some of the issues around whether midwives are empowered enough themselves to be able to offer this kind of service to childbearing women.

VISIONS OF EMPOWERING MIDWIFERY PRACTICE

The fact that some midwives are offering sessions which women and their families find empowering suggests that this is an achievable goal rather than a theory which simply looks good on paper. One student midwife introduced a brief relaxation exercise to seven or eight couples, while they rested in chairs. At the end of the exercise she read a poem entitled *Thirty-Six Weeks* (Grosholz, 1992) which explores the feelings of a woman in the latter weeks of pregnancy towards her baby who is also preparing for birth. The women in the group were of a similar gestation to the woman in the poem and the emotive words expressed were heartfelt. When the group completed the exercise, there wasn't a dry eye in the house and a discussion about how they felt about their babies at this stage in their pregnancy ensued. In a simple way, the student midwife had offered the group an opportunity to examine their feelings and emotions, and possibly to even touch upon the transcendental nature of pregnancy and birth. Pregnancy itself may be considered by the woman to be an intensely spiritual experience. On a physical, psychosocial and spiritual level, it is a rite of passage. We know that encouraging a woman to communicate with her unborn child may have some physical and psychological benefits; we may add to this a spiritual advantage. This felt like a truly empowering experience.

Another midwife who was facilitating a session on infant feeding had a very clearly detailed itinerary of what she was going to present and how she was going to present it. She broke the large group of eighteen into four smaller groups and got one of the sub-groups to identify the benefits of breastfeeding, one the benefits of bottle-feeding, one the disadvantages of breastfeeding and the last the disadvantages of bottle-feeding.

After ten minutes or so the group began to feed back, and an extensive discussion took place. So many of the issues around infant feeding had been raised by this simple exercise and the midwife was able to respond to questions as and when they arose. For example, she was able to demonstrate positioning and attachment from some of the statements that were fed back, and was able to get the group to try out the positions for themselves and say how it felt for them. The issues were not forced and the concerns and queries of the group were bandied around by all of the group members.

One of the reasons that this session stands out is that the matter of addressing infant feeding within a parent education session appears to fill many midwives with varying degrees of concern. In places where the UNICEF Baby Friendly Initiative has been introduced, there does seem to be confusion about what sort of information may be tendered. Concern, which at times appears to border on paranoia, prevents some midwives from even mentioning the word 'bottle', which appears to have led to the charge of 'breastfeeding fascism' (Burchill, 1999) and may have increased the burden of guilt for those women who wish to bottle feed (Battersby, 2000). The UNICEF Baby Friendly Initiative is quite clear within the assessment criteria on how the issue of infant feeding should be addressed by those hospital trusts aiming for Baby Friendly status

(UNICEF, 2003). It suggests that to use time antenatally demonstrating how to make up a bottle of artificial formula is valuable time wasted. What it does not state is that artificial formula cannot be introduced for discussion *per se*, yet it seems, anecdotally at least, that this interpretation is fairly commonplace, leading to the potential disempowerment of women who, for whatever reason, prefer not to breastfeed.

At the end of this particular session, one of the women approached the midwife to offer her thanks. She explained to her that she had been planning to bottle-feed her baby because she felt that so much pressure was being placed on her to breastfeed, that she imagined that she was being set up to fail. However, as a result of the session, she was now going to try breastfeeding because, for the first time, she considered that she had been offered the facts about breastfeeding, objectively and non-judgmentally. In this case, the group leader had truly taken a client-led approach, had let the group take her where they wanted to go, but had nonetheless included the key issues. The group went away feeling a sense of ownership and were much better equipped to make an informed choice about feeding their babies.

Are midwives too oppressed to be liberators?

It is difficult to see midwives offering tools for empowerment such as those described above when they themselves do not feel empowered. It then becomes important to ask questions about the extent to which midwives currently feel they are in control of their own destiny. Or, in other words, whether midwives are too oppressed themselves to be the liberators of childbearing women.

There are many constraints on modern midwifery practice, and midwives are dealing daily with fragmentation of their work, a lack of continuity of working with individual women and massive shortages of midwives with consequent pressures on those who remain in the profession. All but a few lucky (or perhaps empowered?) midwives are working in situations where their working hours and duties are, on the whole, dictated to them. Where midwives have few choices about the way they work, they cannot really be expected to feel as if they are autonomous practitioners. Dare we suggest that the very fact that midwives are not marching on Parliament or all walking out of maternity units together might lead us to the assumption that, with some individual exceptions, midwives are not generally empowered women? If the working conditions of midwives were imposed on a male-dominated profession, we would probably experience national strikes as a result.

Midwives often find themselves in onerous situations where there is deep conflict between the principles of enabling informed choice for women and following hospital policy. While it may be true that there are legal statutes and professional standards which allow women the right to make their own decisions, alongside an expectation that midwives and other attendants will facilitate this, tremendous pressure may be put on the midwife who supports a woman seeking a choice which falls outside of the norm. Midwives may fear the consequences (for both themselves and women) of contradicting hospital policy or professional norms, and, although they might well know that the underpinning regulations are supportive of women's autonomy, they may experience severe social, professional or personal sanctions as a consequence. It is possible that this is one reason why some midwives leading antenatal education sessions feel it is unfair to 'build women's hopes' in offering tools for empowerment; they may not believe that even the most empowered woman can get past the might of the system.

A further consequence of this can be seen in the concept of active disempowerment, where groups who are oppressed themselves then act (whether consciously or unconsciously) to oppress other groups. In other words, the need to control something is experienced by those who have little control themselves. Sadly, this can sometimes be seen in midwifery. Somehow, we need to go about unpacking this in order to enable midwives to realise that the roots of this behaviour may lie in their level of control over their own destiny, and to see the potential consequences of these actions for women and society.

Changing times, changing attitudes: modernism and patriarchy

If we look at empowerment as being about 'holding one's own power', it is possible to surmise some of the reasons why midwives, the vast majority of whom are women, do not see themselves as central to and in control of their own experiences. The loss of our society's reverence for women and their power to create life (Sjoo & Mor, 1997), the centuries of patriarchal dominance (Eisler, 1995) and the positioning of midwifery in some circles as inferior to Western medicine have all taken their toll on the way women feel about their ability to give birth, and the way midwives feel about their ability to help other birthing women. It would therefore be naive to position this debate without reference to the impact which patriarchy has had on society. The modern over-reliance on technology in birth has also played its part.

The changing social norms which birthing women experience have had their own impact on midwifery practice. Even fifty years ago, most women would have had older female relatives nearby to offer information and advice about pregnancy, birth and parenting. However, while there might be a temptation to see women's relative separation from their extended families as detrimental to their empowerment, this is not an assumption that we should make lightly. Sargent and Bascope's (1997) analysis of home birth in Yucatan shows that, in some social settings where traditional midwives and the older women of the community attend births, it is they, rather than the childbearing woman, who tend to hold the authority. In their study, this was especially the case where the woman was giving birth for the first time. Thus such models are not as dissimilar to our own model of medical dominance as we might first imagine, and we should not make the assumption that disempowerment only exists in Western professional settings.

Both antenatal care and antenatal education, as we currently know them, are relative newcomers to the ever-changing role of the midwife. In this age of evidence-based practice, neither of these interventions has been evaluated as effectively as they might, a fact which means that many questions remain about the value of different aspects of these services.

We must also consider the impact of modern society on women's attitudes to birth, not least the way in which some midwives are noticing that a small number of women would prefer not to make choices, having had decisions made for them by others all of their lives. This may be considered a sad consequence of their learned powerlessness or an unreasonable abdication of responsibility, depending on one's perspective. When coupled with the low expectations that some women have of their experience in the maternity services and the fact that women tend to like midwives and don't want to let them down by making unnecessary demands on the service, the stage is set for the continued disempowerment of all concerned.

It is also difficult to have full control over one's destiny in a society where some outcomes – notably death – are seen as socially unacceptable choices. Assisted euthanasia is an illegal act in the UK, and suicide still carries stigma. While this is not to suggest that there are many women who would choose death over medical intervention in birth, there is a need to acknowledge that, in a medical system where safety is the dominant rationality and death is seen both as a failure and something which needs investigation, women's choices are more limited than in a framework where birth is a socio-spiritual rite of passage. All of these things inevitably impact on the empowerment of midwives, the vast majority of whom are also women. While Fahy (2002) proposes that women can be more empowered if the midwife shares knowledge about women's legal rights and the consequences of declining standardised medical care, the pressures on midwives to conform to policies and protocols can make this a thorny path to tread in practice.

Yet, while it may be fair to say that midwives as a social and professional group have, historically, experienced circumstances that may not have been conducive to their empowerment en masse, to say that midwives generally are not empowered is akin to making sweeping statements about the desires or needs of all childbearing women. It is important to remember that, while some midwives may not be – or feel – empowered, there are many others who are. Perhaps a more important line of thinking – to which we shall return – is in considering some of the potential solutions to this situation.

IF NOT MIDWIVES, THEN WHOM?

While midwives may be ideally placed to use their understanding of 'the system' to help women navigate it in enabling their needs to be met, if midwives are not empowered enough to enable the empowerment of childbearing women, it then becomes important to ask whether there is another group better placed to do this. The issue of who is best prepared to deliver antenatal education is an ongoing debate.

Traditionally, women learned about birth and caring for their young from observing their extended families, and caring for younger siblings. The medicalisation of childbirth and the erosion of the extended family heralded the need for 'experts' (usually health professionals) to fill the gap by providing structured antenatal classes to prepare women for the rigours of childbirth and parenting.

In Britain today there are four main providers of antenatal education; those set within the NHS, and within the private, voluntary and other public sectors. The vast majority of antenatal education in the UK is accessed via the NHS and delivered by midwives. It has been suggested that three quarters of midwives are involved in parent education (Kelly, 1998). By contrast, in some countries, such as the US, the independent childbirth educator is part of a vast commercial framework, and woman can shop around to find the classes most suited to their needs. They may explore what Bradley, Lamaze or Birthing from Within (amongst many others) have to offer. The choices are many and diverse.

This diversity is not so apparent in the UK. Private provision is fairly limited and usually quite specialist, for example private yoga sessions and aqua natal classes. Public sector projects, such as SureStart, are often multi-agency. Consequently, they tend to be fragmented and are often short-term projects. They are more common in areas of deprivation as part of health improvement programmes and, while they are a potentially good vehicle for knitting together provision from all sectors, this potential is not always exploited.

Outside the National Health Service, the most familiar provider of antenatal education is the National Childbirth Trust (NCT). This model is provided by a charitable trust and is not a profit making enterprise. NCT teachers are well trained, to diploma level, and have considerable skills and knowledge. However, various people have suggested that the NCT continues to appeal to the middle classes, and promotes middle class attitudes. Although they offer an 'Outreach' policy, offering reduced-cost or free places to those clients who cannot afford to attend their classes, this facility is not well marketed and therefore is not widely accessed.

In their defence, the NCT have attempted and in many cases have managed to successfully establish links with the NHS and now offer workshops for health professionals who go out to the workplace. The Trust also offer a health professionals day during their Annual General Conference each year as well as a health professional page on their website. There may also be a need for the NCT to work more closely with midwives and parents on a more general scale.

It would therefore appear that pregnant women in Britain have a fair chance of accessing antenatal sessions in one guise or another. Yet in spite of this, research over a ten year period has consistently failed to demonstrate that antenatal classes help to prepare women and men for the challenges of early parenting and family life (Coombes & Schonveld, 1992; Holmes & Newburn, 1999). It would seem that parents do not appear to believe that their needs are being met, either in terms of organisation or content. The fact that less than half of all women attend any parent education (Kelly, 1998) may be a reflection of that fact. Those who do attend sessions report that the classes are content-driven and offer few opportunities for questions or discussion. Barclay believes that the problem lies in the fact that there is a huge gulf between the 'professionally defined needs of parents' and what parents actually require (Barclay, conference paper, 1995)

Most, if not all, hospital trusts offer some form of antenatal preparation for parents to be. Some trusts treat parent education as the cornerstone of good midwifery practice, as an opportunity to raise the esteem and confidence of parents to be and provide them with the opportunity to create vital social support networks which may last the rest of their lives. They invest time and effort with parent education high on the professional development agenda. For many others, however, it is viewed at best as an appendage of maternity services and at worst as a necessary evil. In some areas with staffing crises, formal courses have been reduced to two or three sessions or a few hours on a Saturday. Multiparous women may not be invited, because it is felt that they have an existing knowledge of what to expect and therefore will not benefit from what is considered to be a service that is a drain on resources.

Many practising midwives feel ill prepared to take on the mantle of educator in a formal learning and teaching situation. For example, one hospital trust holds 'Tours of the Unit' each weekend, where the pregnant population of the town are invited to turn up and view the maternity unit. The task of having to take what can sometimes be upwards of forty people around the labour and postnatal wards leads to avoidance tactics on a mass scale by the midwives within the unit. Instead of viewing this as an opportunity to facilitate empowerment within the birthing room, they see it as a threatening and fear inducing experience. The issue of how to make this situation manageable is never considered, because the fear of dealing with the ongoing problems clouds judgment and sensibility.

One of the debates which needs to occur within midwifery concerns the question of whether group antenatal education is something which should be a key and core activity carried out by all midwives, or whether this is a specialist role. There are divergent opinions and strong feelings on both sides of this debate. As in the examples at the beginning of this chapter and elsewhere in the book, some midwives and student midwives offer amazing antenatal education sessions which provide all the tools for empowerment that a woman could hope for. Some midwives simply don't feel it is their forte, preferring to work with individual women and couples rather than groups. In an empowered organisation, should midwives be empowered to feel able to decline to undertake this work if they consider that their skills lie elsewhere?

Yet the fact that so many midwives feel so challenged by the role may be about more than a personal dislike of leading groups. Until recently, although it was expected that midwives and health visitors would organise and deliver antenatal education, there was little if any preparation for this eventuality at both pre- and post-registration levels. *The Midwife's Rules and Code of Practice* (Nursing and Midwifery Council, 1998) states that the midwife has an important task in health counselling and education, not only for women but also within the family and community. Yet in 1998, Kelly published survey results which found that 70% of the midwives in the sample rated preparation for such teaching as 'fairly poor' to 'very poor', even though it was recognised that midwives were expected to take on the responsibility of educator as part of their role as defined in statute.

The fact that many midwives felt and continue to feel that they are not equipped with the skills required for what is essentially adult education is a clear problem. The mere thought of standing in front of a group of strangers and being expected to 'teach' them about birth and parenting is anathema. They adopt didactic teaching styles which require a great deal of effort on the part of the practitioner and fail to discover the joy of facilitating a parent education group to enable empowerment.

Midwifery education has recently begun to take parent education seriously, and many of the undergraduate programmes include modules or units of learning dedicated to preparing the students to take on this important role. However, midwives who are already qualified do not generally appear to be as well provided for. This means that those experienced midwives, many of whom are acting as role models to students and more recently qualified midwives, are not offered the opportunity to update their skills and knowledge. This is an area that does require development if we are to provide programmes of parent education that are consistently of a high standard.

The involvement of other health care professionals in antenatal education is sporadic and variable. In some areas, the health visitor leads the classes, embracing the role as part of the public health remit. In others, they are introduced to address specific subject areas such as feeding and parenting. In yet other hospital and community trusts, the health visitor has no input at all.

The physiotherapist is the other health professional who may contribute in some districts, primarily focusing on relaxation and physical preparation for labour. Obstetric physiotherapists are understandably keen to promote their role and to maintain a link with women during this period. However, it is essential that such sessions dovetail with those being delivered by midwives and health visitors which will lead to a joined up and consistent approach.

It may be that the demand for a more empowering approach in parent education will need to emerge from the clients who access the service. An example of this occurred where members of a Maternity Services Liaison Committee decided to explore the availability and quality of antenatal sessions in their specific locality, after their attention was drawn to apparent shortcomings by the local NCT. The findings were not encouraging, with midwives offering very different approaches and varying skills in group facilitation.

As a result of this enquiry, the Head of Midwifery decided to address the problem by making parent education a priority in the strategic planning for the forthcoming year. A parent education co-ordinator was appointed, and regular meetings were held involving all of the stakeholders, including midwives, health visitors, physiotherapists, booking clerks and users. Midwives who were recognised to be skilled and confident in leading classes were identified as key players and were offered the opportunity to attend modules in parenting education at the local university. These midwives were then encouraged to 'buddy' other midwives who were less confident or experienced. One-day workshops were also arranged in collaboration with the university in order to equip any midwives involved in the delivery of parent education with the required skills. The scheme is to be carefully monitored and audited to evaluate the impact on both the midwives and clients. This example demonstrates that when midwifery works in partnership with other agencies and stakeholders, the results can be rewarding.

As this scenario indicates, the answer may lie in a well co-ordinated multi-disciplinary approach which includes a strong user representation. A key health care professional should take the role of coordinator, in order to pull together the other agencies who may be involved in one way or another with the delivery of the service. In order for this to be fully realised, the whole area of antenatal education would need to shed its 'Cinderella' status in the provision of maternity services and adopt a much more prominent profile. This may additionally lead to a more convergent approach to care generally and a greater shared understanding of the contributions of those involved.

Exploring potential solutions

One of the ways in which we could attempt to improve this situation is by looking at further examples of how midwives can be empowered to empower women. 'Walking the talk' is a powerful tool in education. By this we mean offering the student (who may, in this context, be a qualified and experienced midwife) an experience which parallels with that within the parent education setting. When teaching education for parenting in an academic forum, we have used a number of role plays which enable midwives to gain far greater insight into the experience of the parents attending their sessions.

From personal observation we recognise that midwives may be challenged by group members and that they sometimes find this very difficult to deal with. It is this sort of practical problem that disempowers midwives and leads to fear around leading groups. We have used role modelling in order to demonstrate ways of dealing with such group characters. On several occasions during parent education, one of us has led the session whilst the other (who is unknown to the students) plays the part of a disruptive student and sets out to sabotage the session. The facilitator demonstrates how you can usefully deal with a challenging group member and the other students find themselves unwittingly helping the teacher to deal with the troublesome soul present! We 'come clean' at the end of the session, and generally meet with a considerable amount of laughter laced with a good dose of berating. The case has been made and the students have experienced both the facilitator dealing with the problem and have felt what it is to be a group member and how they will frequently jump in and help in such a situation.

Another role play involves getting the students to arrive at the planned venue (usually a university classroom) which is cold, unprepared and unwelcoming. The 'teacher' is equally unwelcoming, brusque and late in arriving. After setting the students some onerous task, the 'teacher' falls out of role and asks the group how they feel.

The group are then moved to a prepared environment where the 'facilitator' greets them, offers them drinks and makes them comfortable. The room is warm and bright and decorated with posters. Books and leaflets are available for them to read and the whole environment contrasts markedly with the soulless room first occupied. This serves as a profound statement about the importance of preparation of the environment. The students usually say immediately that they feel more relaxed and comfortable. They recognise that they feel safer and more willing to learn. The point has been made without any need for wordy academic theory.

As midwife educators we are all too aware of the frustrations that are faced by student midwives in practice areas. We are regularly reminded of the chasm that exists between an evidence-informed curriculum and the lived reality of working in hospitals and other health care settings. This is not a new development but something that has been regularly debated in midwifery education for over a decade (Begley, 2001; Richens, 2002; Phipps 2003).

As teachers on a programme of education designed for qualified midwives, we are in the fortunate position of being able to reach the midwives in practice who may be in a stronger position than student midwives to influence practice and effect change. In the late 1990s we set out to develop a new course that would create midwives who were able to review their own practice, and act as catalysts for change. We were faced with the challenge of creating a course for qualified midwives that could produce practitioners who would effect sustained change in practice as a result of exposure to the educational experience.

The programme was designed to promote excellence in professional practice based upon analysis of practice knowledge and skills. This involved generating new cognitive approaches which help to create a paradigm shift, by encouraging the exploration of individual values, beliefs and philosophies. Central to the philosophy of the programme was the acknowledgement that midwives bring their own personal experiences to the learning experience. The acceptance of the diametrically opposed values of personal versus professional did prove to be an area of conflict for some of those accessing the programme, and for some created considerable dissonance. However, it has been identified that dissonance may pre-empt a change in thinking which will ultimately enable the student to travel with a different view (Mezirow and Associates 1990). The syllabus was therefore structured to enable the experienced practitioner to develop both professionally and personally. The notion of excellence implies the holistic understanding of a subject and relates to outstanding practice. Excellence in practice is important for professional autonomy and personal empowerment. By developing the art of midwifery and furthering knowledge concerning the related sciences, we believed that excellence in practice was achievable.

Learning on the programme was to focus heavily on personal and group interaction and was viewed as a dynamic process which would foster self-awareness and the acquisition of knowledge and skills to improve both the quality of service to mothers, their babies and families, and the development of midwifery. Of particular significance for the course design was App's (1991) emancipatory learning process model. This is an educational model that promotes a dynamic process in which phases may take place simultaneously. It has as its purpose the freeing of people from personal, institutional or environmental forces which may prevent them from seeing new perspectives, from attaining broader and deeper goals and from gaining control in their lives, their communities and beyond.

The course has enjoyed considerable success. It has challenged long-held assumptions and institutionalised activities and practices in post-registration midwifery education (Davies, 2003). In its five-year history, it has produced midwives who appear to be empowered, self aware and motivated, and who have developed strategies to enable them to manage the tension between conflicting forces and elements in practice, which enables them to influence the thoughts and behaviour of others in practice. Many of the students who have completed the course have been involved in some sort of project development. Several have been promoted to senior positions where they are actively facilitating change within their practice areas. The programme illustrates that it is possible to use education as a vehicle for change within midwifery practice using a model and philosophy that could be adopted for use in preparing midwives as facilitators in parent education.

Another potential solution sits within the wider goal of making changes to the system itself. Programs such as De Madres a Madres, based in an inner-city Texan community, have been set up to enable women to provide information and sources of empowerment for each other (McFarlane & Fehir, 1994). Given that birth centres have been clearly demonstrated to promote the empowerment of both childbearing women and their midwives (Spitzer, 1995), the emergent birth centre movement may grow into a potential solution. However, for this to become a reality, we need to find ways to enable the empowerment of more midwives to work towards the goal of a birth centre within reach of every woman – and to believe in their ability to attain that.

CONCLUSIONS

We might consider it is too difficult, in a society which is still patriarchally-focused and constrained by the tenets of modernism, to expect that anywhere near a majority of women can rise above social norms and expectations in order to become empowered. Perhaps the empowerment of women is a much larger task than can be undertaken from within the maternity services alone. Attempting to provide conditions for the empowerment of women in general would, at the very least, require a radical re-positioning of western medicine and the authority it is currently given by society, the dissipation of many of the multinational companies whose advertisements effectively teach women that they are not the experts in how to give birth and feed their babies, the banning of negatively-focused media images and mother and baby magazines and the re-writing of many books.

In suggesting we might continue to attempt to enable the empowerment of midwives themselves, there is a need to acknowledge the authority that 'the system' is given by some midwives, and the impact this has on the way they view their role. There is also a clear need to work towards ways of enabling midwives to practise as the autonomous practitioners that we are, rather than in systems which undermine our own autonomy and that of birthing women.

Yet there are solutions, areas of good practice, and ways in which midwives can – and are – becoming more empowered, and demonstrating excellence in practice. Thus, while it may be fair to say that the balance of the evidence suggests that, generally, and for many reasons, a large proportion of midwives may not currently be empowered enough to effectively empower childbearing women, this is not to suggest that the situation is beyond recovery. Having begun this chapter by being passé, we see no reason not to compound this by ending on a cliché:

Whether you think you can, or you think you can't, you're right.

Attributed to Henry Ford

REFERENCES

Apps J W 1991 Teaching critical thinking. In: Malabar F L Mastering the teaching of adults. Krieger Publishing, Melbourne, Florida, p 95-106

Barclay L 1995 Preparation for parenting: suggestions for improvements based on research. Paper presented at Healthy Families – Healthy Children Conference. International Year of the Family. Sydney, Australia

Battersby S 2000 Breastfeeding and bullying: who's putting the pressure on? Practising Midwife 3(8):36-38

Begley C M 2001 Giving midwifery care: student midwives' views of their working role. Midwifery 17(1):24-34

Burchill J 1999 Breastfeeding sucks. Guardian 12 May 1999. Online. Available: http:// www.guardian.co.uk/ parents/story/0,3605,296666,00.html

Coombes G, Schonveld A 1992 Life will never be the same again. Health Education Authority, London

Davies L 2003 A feminist approach to midwifery education. In: Stewart M (ed) Pregnancy, birth and maternity care: feminist perspectives. Elsevier, Oxford, p 154

Davis-Floyd R 1992 Birth as an Ameriacan Rite of Passage. University of California Press, Berkeley, CA

Eisler R 1995 The chalice and the blade, 2nd edn. HarperCollins, New York

Fahy K 2002 Reflecting on practice to theorise empowerment for women using Foucault's concepts. Australian Journal of Midwifery 15(1):5-13

Flint C 1990 Power over birth: its importance for women. Obstetrics and Gynaecology Product News Spring:16-17

Grosholz E 1992 Eden. John Hopkins University Press, Baltimore

Holmes K, Newburn M 1999 NCT services – birth, becoming a mother and baby feeding. New Generation Digest October :18-20

Kelly S 1998 Parent education survey. RCM Midwives Journal 1(1):23-25

McFarlane J, Fehir J 1994 De madres a madres: a community, primary health care program based on empowerment. Health Education Quarterly 21(3):381-394

Merali I 2001 Advancing women's reproductive and sexual health through empowerment and human rights. Journal of Obstetrics and Gynaecology 23(8):694-700

Mezirow J and Associates 1990 Fostering critical reflection in adulthood: a guide to transformative and emancipatory learning. Jossey Bass, San Francisco

Phipps F M 2003 Educating midwives: where do we go from here? Midwifery Matters 96:12-16

Priest J, Schott J 1994 Leading antenatal classes. Butterworth Heinemann, London

Rappaport J 1984 Studies in empowerment: introduction to the issue. Prevention in Human Services 3:1-7

Richens Y 2002 Are midwives using research evidence in practice? British Journal of Midwifery 10(10):11-16

Sargent C, Bascope G 1997 Ways of knowing about birth in three cultures. In: Davis-Floyd R E, Sargeant C F (eds) Childbirth and authoritative knowledge: cross-cultural perspectives. University of California Press, Berkeley, p 183-208

Sjoo M, Mor B 1997 The great cosmic mother; rediscovering the religion of the earth. Harper and Row, San Fransisco

Spitzer M C 1995 Birth centers. Economy, safety, and empowerment. Journal of Nurse-Midwifery 40(4):371-375

Nursing and Midwifery Council 1998 The midwives' rules and code of practice. Online. Available: www.nmc-uk.org/nmc/main/publications/midwives.pdf

Too S-K 1996 Do birthplans empower women? A study of their views. Nursing Standard 10(31):33-37

UNICEF 2003 Online. Available: http://www.babyfriendly.org.uk/guid-ant.asp#group)

Wallerstein N 1992 Powerlessness, empowerment and health promotion program. American Journal of Health Promotion 6(3):197-205

Chapter 6

Innovative Practice in Birth Education
Birmingham Women's Hospital Birth Ideas Workshops

Julie Foster

What does antenatal education that really enables women to choose for themselves how they would like to give birth look like? Recent research suggests that the environment of birth is critical in influencing the way in which women behave in labour, and in promoting fear, tension and increased pain. Birth Ideas Workshops take birth education into the delivery room. They familiarise women and their supporters with the environment, and show them how to adapt it to assist rather than hinder them in achieving a birth experience that enriches their lives. The attitude of midwives towards the use of so-called 'alternative positions' and upright, active birth is critical in determining whether or not they can lead Birth Ideas Workshops which will demystify the birth environment for women. It may be that midwives also need educating not only in how to run Birth Ideas Workshops, but also so that they can regain their confidence in the philosophy that underpins them.

(Editors' note)

> *We are the torchbearers of truth, the tellers of tales of beautiful birth, the weavers of courageous empowering visions to set before the women and families we serve.*
>
> Edmonds, 2003

As childbirth educators working within the NHS, we are entrusted with the momentous task of helping childbearing women and their families to acquire knowledge, problem solve, develop self help skills for labour, and to grow in confidence that nature can be trusted when it comes to birth. This may well be our aspiration, but how many of us find the back up we and our clients need for such a philosophy on the delivery ward? If there is no such back-up, are we guilty of setting up our clients with unrealistic hopes and expectations and then, metaphorically speaking, throwing them to the lions? Do we talk of control, empowerment, normality and confidence and then herd the women into a clinical delivery room where they will have little or no control over their own labours and births and where intervention is the norm?

There can be no doubt that preparation for birth in its many guises is an influential factor in determining the way in which labour, birth and early parenting are perceived, approached and actualised. Birth experiences that fall short of women's expectations, like any other significant event in life, have the potential to undermine or even devastate their confidence and sense of identity. The majority of midwives would argue that we should not be censoring the information that we give to expectant parents, in order to protect ourselves or any other health care professionals. However, we can rarely escape the medical model of childbirth, nor the environment and culture in which we are challenged to operate as 'experts in the normal'.

Are we thinking as autonomous practitioners, able to recognise where our 'uncensored' information may have become tainted by our over zealous and curative birth culture? Are we empowered and confident enough to challenge orthodoxy that is clearly not in the interests of women? Are we teaching women compliance and dependency, trademark factors in the demise of normality, or are we teaching them how to be confident and challenging consumers of the maternity services?

As Robertson (2002) points out, midwife educators are employed to prepare women for delivery in our hospitals and generally expected to explain policies and procedures rather than discuss options that many hospitals would rather not provide. Similarly, clinical midwives are employed to care for women within those policies and are expected to carry out procedures according to the biomedical model of birth. As educators we can tell women about normal birth and how to achieve it, but we cannot guarantee that their caregivers will share our ideals or support them in their choices. A woman's confidence, strength and ability to give birth are enhanced or destroyed by her birth attendants and the birth environment. This presents us with a dilemma: how do we bridge the gap between women's expectations and our experience?

This chapter will focus on why traditional delivery suite tours often do more harm than good, and will present Birth Ideas Workshops as an alternative, innovative model of practice that has the potential to impact not only on the way in which couples approach and experience labour and birth, but on the birth environment and culture as a whole.

TRADITIONAL DELIVERY SUITE TOURS – WHAT IS WRONG WITH THEM?

At Birmingham Women's Hospital (BWH), the tour of delivery suite was a daunting task. Every Sunday there would be a discussion as to who was free to meet the group, which invariably ended with a very reluctant midwife being allocated the task. While few would argue that it is helpful for couples to gain an insight into the delivery suite environment, the content and process of our tours were doing women a disservice. Feedback from both staff and couples was overwhelmingly negative, yet we continued under the assumption that lack of resources meant lack of ability to improve the service.

Student midwives were 'shown the ropes' which included taking the bed apart to demonstrate how it looks in preparation for lithotomy. We handed around forceps, ventouse cups, amnihooks and fetal scalp electrodes, and demonstrated how the resuscitaire works while explaining that babies often need help with their first breaths. Couples arrived in droves each week to see the inside of delivery suite and alleviate some of their fears, yet often they left our department not only in fear of the rooms but also in fear of their lives!

The impetus for change came from a visit by Gina (not her real name) who made an appointment to be shown around delivery suite with her mother. Gina had attended a delivery suite tour the previous week and had been traumatised by the experience. This is her account of that tour:

My husband and I were told just to turn up on Sunday at 2pm. When we got to the hospital, after a nightmare trying to park, there were about 30 people waiting in the reception area. They were all heavily pregnant, so we knew we were in the right place! Then a young midwife came out to meet us. She obviously wasn't expecting so many of us, because she looked terrified. She rounded us all up and began trying to explain about the toilets and so on, but most of us couldn't hear what she was saying, even though she was trying to shout to those of us standing at the back. She led us through the hospital to the delivery suite. When we got to the main entrance, she stopped to tell us something about security. We were blocking the corridor and a pregnant woman who looked in pain was wheeled through the middle of our crowd and into the delivery suite. Poor woman. I know you can expect to lose your dignity but I hope I don't have such a large audience when I go into labour. We couldn't all get into a delivery room at the same time, so half of the group had to stand outside while the midwife went to ask if there was someone else who could look after us. After about ten minutes, a second midwife arrived and took us into another room. We all had to stand around the bed. There was equipment everywhere. The midwife asked us what we wanted to know. I had a list of questions to ask, but nobody said anything and I was too embarrassed to read my list out. I think we were all in awe of the room, trying to imagine what it was going to be like when our turn came. She began to show us the machine for when the baby isn't breathing and she passed around a knitting needle thing for when your waters don't break. We were told how to use the bell to call the midwife if we needed help and then to my horror, one of the men asked about forceps. The midwife produced a set of giant metal forceps and the group were told to pass them around. Apparently, they are quite safe and cradle the baby's head on the way out, but I can't get that image out of my mind. I didn't even look at the rest of the stuff she showed us. My husband did and he thought it was good to know what to expect so it's not a shock when the time comes, but I could feel my knees going to jelly. The room looked really cold and unwelcoming and to be honest, I'm worried sick that I won't be able to cope. My husband tells me that all the medical stuff is important and that it saves lives, and I can see that. I don't want you to think that I don't appreciate that it is there for when it's needed. I would just rather not have to see it all before it's needed. My mom said I should ask to come in on my own and see a midwife so that she could explain it all to me properly and maybe, you know, help me to stop worrying a bit.

To summarise Gina's concerns:
- The tour was badly organised and oversubscribed.
- The midwife seemed out of her depth and did not project confidence.
- Gina felt unwelcome and in the way.
- She felt too embarrassed to ask any questions.
- The environment was cold and unfriendly.
- The bed and equipment were the focal points of the tour.
- Gina was frightened by the forceps/instruments/lack of privacy.
- She was worried about saying anything in case she was seen as 'ungrateful'.

Other evaluations of the traditional tour reflected Gina's concerns, as did evaluations completed by the midwives running them.

A frequent topic of conversation in the coffee room on the delivery suite was the powerlessness we feel as midwives to be autonomous practitioners. However, after a couple of hours spent with Gina, it was clear that we had to take at least some of the blame for perpetuating the medicalisation of birth. Her second visit to the hospital helped formulate the following questions:
- Why do couples want to see the delivery rooms?
- What do they want to know?
- What do they need to know?
- What do we tell them?
- What do they discover for themselves?
- What kind of birth are we preparing them for?
- What is our philosophy?
- What are our goals?

Any midwife showing parents around the delivery suite would have found it difficult to answer these questions in the absence of clearly defined goals or an underpinning philosophy for the tour. Couples are frequently advised to prepare themselves for birth by familiarising themselves with the environment in which the birth is scheduled to take place. For most couples, the tour will be the first contact they have with the delivery suite. It is during this visit that fear is reinforced or diminished. It is here that the good work of childbirth educators can be enhanced or destroyed.

Couples tell us they *want to know* what the delivery suite is like, how to get there, the procedures on arrival, who will greet them, what facilities are available and what to bring in. Yet much of this information can probably be found in our hospital guidebooks, while too little time is spent on helping them to focus on the experience of birth, the birth environment and their roles within it.

What they *need to know* is that they are not just visitors to our work place; they do not have to fit in around us. They have the right to negotiate and to adapt the environment where possible to fit in with their requirements. They need a clear understanding that the vast majority of uncomplicated pregnancies result in uncomplicated births and that the vast majority of the equipment on display will have no use in their labour and birth. They do not necessarily need to know what the equipment is for, but they do need to know how to question its use. They need to know how to focus on their internal resources as well as the external resources, and use them both.

What do we tell them? We tell them what we told Gina. And just as Gina did, most couples will deduce from such a tour that they will be constrained by a clinical environment more suited to having a leg amputated than to giving birth, and that they are at the mercy of a whole host of instruments and interventions in the interests of safety.

So, just what kind of birth are we preparing our couples for? Well, of course, we are preparing them for a good outcome! But just what is a good outcome? Vaginal birth? Pain free? No stitches? Becoming obsessed with the 'right' way to give birth or the 'right' way to feel about the birth experience is counterproductive. By so doing, we are telling women to 'perform or fail'; we are initiating the fear – tension – pain cycle that is so unhelpful to labouring women and which makes intervention more likely. Birth is as unpredictable as it is fascinating; no amount of preparation can guarantee a given outcome, and as Niven (1992) points out, objective facts do not prepare people for a subjective experience. What women and their partners need first and foremost is a basic understanding of what is happening during labour, confidence to trust the power and innate wisdom of the woman's body to birth unaided, and the opportunity to explore and heed the messages and signs that the women's bodies will undoubtedly give them. The mothers need 'permission' and freedom to work with their bodies in our alien and bustling birth environments in order that they may find their own creative solutions. Ultimately, they need a tool kit of skills to help them find their way through labour, birth and any unexpected event which arises.

BIRTH IDEAS WORKSHOP (BIW)

Following the meeting with Gina, a working party was set up to look at how best to address the problems arising from the traditional tours. The working party comprised motivated midwives with a keen interest in normalising the birth process (birth change agents), representatives from the NCT and Active Birth, and users of the service. Aims and objectives were clarified:

BIW Aims and objectives

Aims

- To enable couples to feel confident within the hospital birth environment
- To empower and prepare couples emotionally, psychologically and physically for their labour and birth experience

Objectives

- Explore individuals' fears
- Explore and evaluate the birth environment
- Explore an alternative perspective on pain
- Review the normal physiological process of birth
- Explain the three 'p's: power, passage and passenger
- Explore and discuss partners' role
- Practise a variety of self-help techniques
- Practise a variety of positions for labour and birth that will enhance the normal physiology
- Practise creating couples'/women's own 'safe environment'

BIWs were implemented in December 2001. They incurred little extra cost or resources. The biggest challenge was to change the attitudes of staff whose practice over the years had become entrenched in the medical model. However, with a dedicated team of birth change agents and strong management support, BIWs have now become a permanent feature at BWH.

The format

Length and timing of sessions

BIW sessions are held every Saturday and Sunday at 13.30 during the staff handover period and last for approximately two hours. Due to their popularity and the high number of births at BWH, it was initially necessary to run 'overspill' sessions during the week. However, the parent education team have now incorporated the BIW session into their evening courses, so freeing weekends for couples who do not attend any other parent education.

Venue

Whenever possible, a delivery suite room is used for the BIWs. Having the opportunity to discuss fears and participate in practical activities within the actual birth environment helps to bring the session alive, aids retention of information given and demystifies the clinical setting. The room is always exactly as the couples will find it on admission. Inevitably, there are times when all rooms are occupied, and the parent education room has to be used instead. The BIW session can be satisfactorily simulated here with photographs of the delivery room used to create the context.

Group size

A maximum of five women and their partners are invited to each BIW session. Keeping the numbers low is imperative because of venue capacity and:
- To create an informal environment in which attendees feel able to express their fears and concerns
- To facilitate discussion/questions
- To allow a more individualised approach
- To allow participation in practical aspects of the session.

Clientele

The workshops are open to all clients, regardless of parity, who have completed 34 weeks of pregnancy and are anticipating a vaginal birth. Audit revealed that 56% of those attending BIWs had not enrolled on any other parent education courses. This reflects the motivation of couples to see the delivery suite prior to their labours, and presents us with an opportunity to reach many clients with parent education who would otherwise 'slip through the net'.

Bookings

Information about the BIWs and parent education services in general is given to all women at booking. They receive a form to complete and return to the Parent Education Department before 24 weeks of pregnancy, stating their preferences for courses. The majority of women book through this system. Appointments are then loaded onto a database and letters sent out to women with dates and times of all sessions they wish to attend. This facilitates the audit process as well as being a seamless method of booking.

Staffing   Midwives from all areas are expected to facilitate the BIWs. A rota system operates whereby delivery suite and each ward area take turns to provide a midwife to run a session. The rota is circulated twelve months in advance, so that each area knows exactly when they will have to provide cover. Having midwives from each department working to the same format and delivering the same content reduces the risk of conflicting information. However, there is always scope for individual teaching styles and creativity is encouraged.

Training   Midwives are expected to observe at least one BIW before leading a workshop of their own. Training sessions are available to staff during the mid-week handover periods. The Parent Education Team provides regular updates for all staff and newcomers to the Trust. A comprehensive, step-by-step folder is available for reference in each area.

Resources
- Delivery room (parent education room as back-up)
- Delivery bed
- Length of entonox tubing
- Fetal doll with placenta and amniotic sac
- Pelvis
- 'Post it' stickers
- Birthing balls/beanbags/pillows
- Floor mats
- Extra chairs
- Evaluation forms/pens
- Handouts (optional).

Birth Ideas Workshop: Format and content

Greeting the group   The parents are asked to meet in the hospital coffee shop from where the allocated midwife collects them. The coffee shop is quite small, and parents will often strike up conversation before the BIW begins. The midwife has a list of the people expected to attend and greets them by name.

The midwife then takes the couples on the journey that they will make when coming into hospital, explaining
- Where to park
- Out of hours access to delivery suite
- Restaurant facilities
- Visiting times
- Telephones/toilets/cashiers
- Orientation to the delivery suite/ward areas.

Questions are encouraged.

Delivery suite Outside the delivery suite, access and admission procedures are explained and attention is drawn to the security system and the importance of maintaining a secure environment. The aim is not to alarm parents, but to reassure them that their safety is paramount and that they have a role to play in this also. They are encouraged to ask to see identity badges and not to hold doors open for unknown persons.

The general layout of delivery suite is explained, and where possible, the shift leader introduces herself to the group, outlining her role. Couples are told that there are three shifts in any 24-hour period so it is possible that they may have more than one midwife caring for them in labour. The group is shown where the toilets, refreshments and waiting areas are.

Admissions The group are shown the admissions rooms and the triage system is explained. The three possible routes out of admissions are discussed i.e. home, to the ward or to a delivery room. This is an opportunity to mention the importance of staying at home as long as possible in the absence of any complication, and telephoning ahead so that staff can offer advice on self-help techniques and prepare for their arrival.

Delivery room

Icebreaker The group is then shown into a delivery room. One person is given a pad of post-it stickers. The midwife explains that the parents will be left alone for five minutes. They are encouraged to explore the room, look inside cupboards and behind curtains. Each group member is asked to place a sticker on an item that they would like explained. Although the aim is not to discuss individual items of equipment, placement of the stickers gives away lots of clues as to what the group are anxious about and explanations can easily be built into the session. Once they have placed the post-its, they are asked to come outside and collect a chair. This activity has proved to be an excellent icebreaker. The couples, surprised to be left alone in the room, have to communicate in order to share the stickers and have fun doing so.

After five minutes, the group will usually have emerged. If not, the midwife begins to carry the chairs in. In most delivery rooms, the bed is the focal point, so the chairs are placed in a semi-circle around it. Once seated, the group is asked to chat to the couple next to them. They are asked to find out the following:

- Names
- How many weeks pregnant they are and whether this is their first baby
- One positive thing about the pregnancy so far
- One thing they are not looking forward to about labour.

Where there are uneven numbers, the facilitating midwife joins in. This enables the couples to interact and share with each other common joys and fears associated with childbirth.

Introductions

After five minutes, the facilitating midwife takes her place in the centre of the group, preferably sitting on the bed. This position is strategic. Later in the session, the group will be encouraged to think about how subtle non-verbal actions such as this often communicate professional dominance.

Ground rules are set, the group is asked to turn off mobile phones and invited to take a comfort break at any time. A tray of cold drinks is ready in the room. People are encouraged to ask questions and actively participate throughout the session. The midwife introduces herself, telling the parents something about her professional role and something personal. The aims of the session are outlined and parents are told that they will be looking at *power, passenger* and *passage*. The group is then invited to share the information they have gained while talking to each other. Often the men and women will introduce each other.

The positive experiences that the group members share vary enormously. The negatives however, rarely differ from the list below.

Women	*Men*
● Pain	● Seeing partner in pain
● Coping with labour	● Feeling powerless to help
● Things going wrong	● Things going wrong

Invariably, the main concern is fear of pain. This leads into the main body of the session.

SESSION CONTENT

Part 1 – Power

Key questions
- Why does it hurt to have a baby?
- What would happen if there were no pains?

Pain is normally a sign that something is wrong. In childbirth, it's a sign that everything is right! Explain why labour hurts, what is happening to the women's bodies, how contractions start, peak and end. Encourage the group to think about what is happening at the peak of a contraction, and how pain is productive and positive (as opposed to other sorts of pain they have experienced).

- How do you cope with pain normally? (find a comfortable position, heat, darkness, massage, music etc.)

- Will the environment you are in now inhibit you from using these tried and tested coping mechanisms?
- How might the birth environment affect the way you cope with pain during labour?
- What factors might make the pain seem more intense and unmanageable? (fear, anxiety, tension, lack of support, hostile environment)
- When you are anxious, you instinctively tense your muscles. How do you think that affects your body's ability to birth your baby?
- How can you work with or against your body to birth your baby?

A woman in fear, either of the birth process, the pain or the environment, will instinctively protect her baby by keeping it safely inside her womb. The group are reminded that birth has evolved over thousands of years and is undoubtedly the most powerful and awesome creative force known to us. Magnificently designed and innately equipped, women have the wisdom and the ability to give birth and babies to be born. Yet over a number of decades, we as professionals and as a society have taught women to fear birth by interfering with this finely tuned, physiological process, constraining women's creativity and undermining their inherent wisdom about how to give birth.

Encourage the group to think of examples of how fear affects them.

Fear has become the major driving force behind every decision a woman makes. We have denied women their primitive animal instinct to birth in a dark, safe and private environment and instead, we tell them what to do and how to do it and assure them that modern technology will come to the rescue when their bodies fail. Fear dictates the 'management' of birth on our labour wards.

By sharing these thoughts with the group, the midwife encourages participants to think about where the power of birth lies and where it should lie. One way of giving back some power to the labouring woman and her companion is to arm them with a list of questions that they can use in any unexpected situation that might arise during labour:

- What is the reason for the procedure?
- Why is it necessary?
- What are the advantages and disadvantages for me and my baby?
- Is there anything else I could try first?
- What happens if I wait for a couple of hours?
- What happens if I decide I do not want to have this procedure at all?

The group is reminded of the role of the shift leader and encouraged to ask for a second opinion if in doubt. The partner's role as advocate is raised and discussed at this point.

In part one, the midwife aims to decrease the fear of pain in childbirth by explaining that if women work with their bodies and embrace the uncomfortable sensations rather than fight them, they will be more relaxed and their contractions more effective. Most parents will never have questioned why it hurts to have a baby, nor thought about the productive and powerful nature of contractions. Having recognised that pain is nature's way of helping them to make and mark the transition from being somebody's child to being somebody's parent, many couples report a sense of excitement about the impending labour and birth.

Holding the session in the delivery room enables the facilitator to refer the group to aspects of the environment that may inhibit their sense of control, whilst suggesting ways to personalise the room.

Part 2 – Passenger

Key questions

- What role does the baby play in labour and delivery?
- What position does baby need to be in for labour to progress smoothly? (OA vs. OP etc.)
- What factors affect the position of your baby? (e.g. sedentary lifestyle, posture, comfortable furniture, dishwashers etc.)
- What can you do to encourage your baby into the LOA position?
- How will your baby let you know that he/she needs more room?
- How can you tell if your baby is in the wrong position?

Part 2 of the session is heavily indebted to Jean Sutton's work (2001) on optimal fetal positioning. The midwife explains to the group that it is important to adapt their lifestyle wherever possible to encourage an occiput anterior (OA) position, but it is not a disaster if their baby is occiput posterior (OP) prior to birth. Most babies will get themselves into the correct position during the labour if the mother's position allows them to do so.

Following a demonstration with the pelvis, the women are asked to use the fetal model to work out what position they think their baby may be in according to how they are now sitting and taking into account the effect of gravity. Using the same chair/beanbag they are sitting on, they are then asked to demonstrate a position which will be more conducive to optimal fetal positioning. This enables the midwife to evaluate their understanding. The group is encouraged to suggest small changes they can make to their lifestyle that will encourage optimal fetal positioning, for example, avoiding bucket seats, lying on their left side instead of reclining on the sofa and practising cat arches when the baby is active. A handout is provided.

Part 3 – Passage   *Key questions*

- How does your position during labour and delivery affect:
    - Baby's position?
    - The space available for baby to negotiate the birth canal?
    - The length, strength and efficiency of your contractions (power)?
    - The length of the first and second stages of labour?
    - Your sense of control, participation and achievement?
    - Your birthing partner's role?
- How can you use your mobility to enhance labour and delivery (pelvic tilt, gravity, rhombus of michaelis)?

The entonox tubing, found in all delivery rooms, is an invaluable aid for demonstrating what happens to the birth canal when a woman is in a supported sitting position. The group are asked what would happen to a ping-pong ball (representing the baby's head) placed inside the tubing when the tubing is vertical (equivalent of the mother being in an upright position) and when it is curved in a U bend (equivalent of the mother being in a supported sitting position). This is a very effective teaching aid and many couples comment on their evaluations how clearly it gets the point across.

Using the model of the fetus complete with amniotic sac and placenta enables the facilitator to demonstrate the effectiveness of contractions in OA and OP and the effects of gravity and the mother's position. The use of the pelvic tilt to maximise the power of the contraction by bringing the baby directly onto the cervix can also be shown. The midwife explains the first and second stages and encourages the group to think about the distinct purpose of each and how women's bodies signal to them what is happening.

The couples are invited to practise optimal positions using the birthing ball, beanbags, and the bed as props. Partners are encouraged to move the bed to one side to maximise the floor space and potential for mobility, and place mattresses on the floor. The aim is to enable the group to feel confident and at ease to alter the room as they choose.

The midwife's role is to help the group discover suitable positions for themselves and ensure that they adhere to the principles of safety. The women are encouraged to think about how their perception of the baby's weight alters in each position they take up, so helping them to link the fetal position with their own. The role of the partners is addressed throughout, with tips on how they can be actively involved in the labour. They work with the women to find ways of supporting them in each position and massage techniques are demonstrated to help them ease the women's discomfort.

By this point in the session, the group has usually forgotten about the equipment and their post-it stickers, and when asked if they still require explanations, often say that they would rather not know! It is tremendously rewarding to enter the delivery room with an anxious group of expectant parents who want to know what all the wires and machines are for, and to be with them at the end of the session when they are so positive about how they will approach labour that they no longer see the equipment as having a major role.

IMPACT OF BIW AT BWH

The first 100 couples who attended BIWs were asked to complete an evaluation form about the delivery suite environment. Their comments were overwhelmingly negative. These were presented to management as powerful evidence from the users of the service about the need to alter the clinical environment and make it more appropriate for birth. It was agreed that changes were needed

We approached our local TV station and presented them with a 'changing rooms' opportunity. They were delighted to be involved and offered us top designers and £2000 for the project, which involved transforming two delivery rooms and the waterbirth room. Trust management matched this amount. Given the media involvement, several local companies were willing to provide their services free of charge. Our budget therefore remained largely untouched. On completion, the rooms were showcased on the local news and we subsequently received phone calls from other local businesses wanting to sponsor a room of their own.

The make-over project enabled us to look at changing the position of the bed and removing the workstation. This caused considerable controversy. The medical staff were not happy to have the bed against the wall as their access would be restricted. We compromised. The bed was placed diagonally in the corner of the room, thereby enabling access but making it less prominent. Removing the workstations also proved to be a problem. Many of the midwives complained that they would have nowhere to write their notes and to sit with their notes on their laps would cause them backache. Yet the positioning of the workstations in modern delivery rooms tends to require the midwife to turn her back to the labouring woman, thereby diminishing communication. Another compromise was found here by introducing a stylish cupboard on wheels that could also be used as a workstation.

For the first six months, birth change agents – midwives involved in the BIWs – ran the weekly sessions. This was to allow midwives from all clinical areas to observe a session and participate, before they were rolled out. Various problems were encountered. Many midwives refused to run the sessions. One senior midwife asked, 'Why should I teach something I don't believe in?' Another commented that, 'It's not my job to crawl around the floor catching babies'. Yet another said, 'If I'm allocated to run the session, I will just go off sick'. These were disheartening comments, but not entirely unexpected. Any change is a challenge that requires courage and is not without risk.

Training sessions were held by the birth change agents, and all midwives were invited to attend. Just four midwives, but 15 student midwives, attended the first session. We were heavily criticised for presuming to know more about facilitating birth than our colleagues. This was undoubtedly a smokescreen to hide the real issue which was that many midwives had never seen or undertaken a delivery in any other position than supported sitting, and although women often requested alternative positions, they would always find a reason for the woman to get onto the bed. They were also afraid that if anything were to go wrong at the birth, they would be criticised for not 'doing it properly'. If they were not confident in facilitating women's choices for optimal fetal positioning, they felt the need to work with a midwife who had more confidence. The overall effect of the BIW training sessions and the workshops themselves was to open up a refreshing and long overdue debate within the unit, and to highlight an urgent need for further training.

Birth Ideas Workshops – Audit findings

Following ten months of regular BIW sessions, a retrospective survey of 300 women was undertaken, 150 who had attended BIWs and 150 who had not. Both groups comprised 110 primiparous women and 40 multiparous. We audited methods of pain relief and positions used by the women for birth for the period between December 2001 and September 2002.

In the previous two year period, the percentage of women giving birth in 'alternative positions' (i.e. standing, kneeling, squatting, all fours, left lateral) was as follows:

- 2000 = 5.9%
- 2001 = 7.4%

Among the women who *did not* attend a BIW within the audit period, the percentage of deliveries in alternative positions was 7.28%.

Among the women who *did* attend a BIW within the audit period, the percentage of deliveries in alternative positions was 36.2%. (Figure 6.1)

The increase in the number of women giving birth other than on their backs was dramatic. While other variables may have influenced the results, it is not unreasonable to presume that the increase was due to the fact that BIW attendees were shown where the beanbags, birthing balls and mattresses are kept, how to use them and had developed an understanding of the importance of mobility in labour and optimal positioning for birth.

Even more striking than this finding is the number of women opting for an epidural among the BIW attendees. (Figure 6.2)

Figure 6.1
Comparison of delivery
positions among BIW attendees
and non-attendees Dec 2001 –
Sep 2002

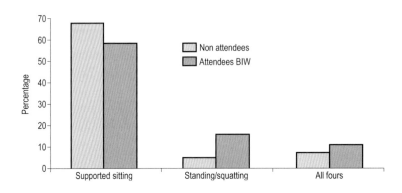

Figure 6.2
Comparison of epidural rates
among BIW attendees and non-
attendees Dec 2001 – Sep 2002

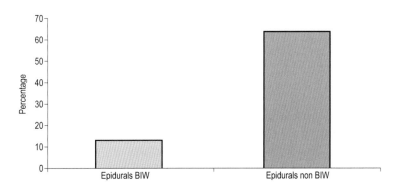

Sixty per cent of non-attendees opted for an epidural, and only 13% of those who had been to a Birth Ideas Workshop. Medical forms of analgesia are not discussed during the workshop. Any couples who have questions on epidurals or pethidine are seen separately at the end of the session. We cannot prove conclusively that BIWs were responsible for the dramatic difference in epidural rates. Yet there certainly seems to be a link and readers are invited to draw their own conclusions.

CONCLUSION

BIWs have transformed the way in which women and their partners are introduced to the delivery suite environment and ultimately, to the way in which they prepare for and approach labour and birth. At BWH, we have seen a critical mass of women coming through the system, who know what they want and are asking for it. We have seen a change in attitude among midwives, even those who were initially resistant to change and who have now made the effort to reflect on their practice and update their skills so that they can facilitate women in their choices.

Of the three hundred women we asked 'Would you recommend the Birth Ideas Workshop to a friend?', 100% said 'Yes'.

- 'Very useful and informative. I liked the direct, honest approach.'
- 'Thank you! I learnt more from the last two hours than I did from having my last three babies.'
- 'I'm actually looking forward to the birth now, which I never thought I'd say.'
- 'I know how I can help my wife now and I'm not so worried about fainting.'
- 'I feel cheated – in my day we had to lie on the bed and take it, but this way makes so much more sense.' (Granny)

REFERENCES

Edmonds J 2003 Quote of the week. Online. Available: www.midwiferytoday.com

Niven C 1992 Psychological care for families before, during and after birth. Butterworth Heinemann, Oxford

Robertson A 2002 Education for informed choice. Online. Available www.acegraphics.com

Sutton J 2001 Let birth be born again. Birth Concepts, UK

Chapter 7

Best Practice in Antenatal Education

Traditional antenatal classes are known to be attractive to only a small section of the pregnant community. Women who do not speak English, who belong to a different culture from the indigenous one, who are poor or ill educated, or very young do not choose to attend classes where they fear they will feel out of place or appear ignorant or be stigmatised. Some women live in isolated areas where classes are simply not available. While the desire to reach out to these women is strong in many hospital and community Trusts, it is not always clear what strategies would be the most successful. This chapter looks at seven examples of excellent practice in the field of antenatal education, providing models of educational and support services for women in a variety of often difficult circumstances.

(Editors' note)

Improving Services for Women of South Asian Heritage

Sheena Byrom and Clare Harding

Unwitting racism can arise because of a lack of understanding, ignorance or mistaken beliefs. It can arise from well intentioned but patronising actions. It can arise from unfamiliarity with behaviour or cultural traditions of people or families from ethnic minority communities. It can arise from stereotyping. (Macpherson, 1999)

Queen's Park Hospital Maternity Unit, Blackburn serves a culturally diverse population, and currently 32.2% of the 3,500 annual births are to women of Asian heritage, with 70% coming from Pakistan. Research informs us that women of Pakistani origin want information, communication and continuity from the maternity services (Richens, 2003), reflecting the needs of Caucasian populations. This client group

Figure 7.1
Perinatal mortality rate

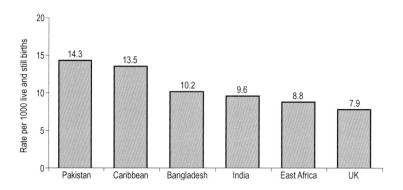

is less likely to access appropriate services, resulting in unacceptable levels of maternal and perinatal deaths. Women from India, Bangladesh and Pakistan have three times the risk of maternal death compared with white women (CEMD, 2001), and up to twice the perinatal mortality rate of Caucasian women (ONS, 1999), (Figure 7.1).

In Blackburn, women of Asian heritage were not accessing services, particularly antenatal education. Focus groups were held in the community, using well-respected and locally known midwives and link workers to invite and transport women. (Women and families are now invited three times yearly to a local venue to discuss their 'journey' through maternity services. Their comments are noted and discussed with managers, and responses are sent back to the attendees. The process feeds into the Trust's user involvement strategy.)

A significant proportion of the women attending had little or no English, so previously their voice was rarely heard. Participants initially praised the services, but when asked how they could be improved, identified the following:

- the lack of a local venue
- cultural issues
- the needs of older children.

As a result, an appropriately-timed drop-in service for antenatal and postnatal mothers has been developed in a local community centre, with a crèche (Payne & Fleming, 2002). Two Asian mothers and a link worker have now been trained to lead the group. They identified their strengths, as well as their needs (practical methods for running the group, communication and listening skills, and dealing with difficult situations). Needs were met through a 20-hour course, with 10 hours subsequent supervision to give support and discuss problems. Midwifery input is provided by midwives who have received training in facilitating client-led education, through a 6-day English National Board approved course.

The midwives identified their aims for the group as:

- making it client-led
- addressing inequalities
- promoting positive images of midwifery
- promoting the health and wellbeing of the women
- empowerment of the women.

Mothers identified theirs as:

- access to multi-agency information on pregnancy, birth and childcare in the early years
- sharing and debriefing experiences
- meeting their social needs (relaxation, meeting other mothers, gaining support)
- empowerment (through information, time for themselves, and making mothers feel valued).

Sessions are unstructured and totally client-led, with multi-agency input. There is an emphasis on sharing knowledge, and mixing leisure with learning. Comments from mothers using the service support this:

> ... Well I think they [Asian women] need a bit of an outing rather than just talking ... so they know the places to go so they are independent as well if their husband's not there for them. They can take their children out ... because they're stuck indoors they don't know where to go and how to get out of the house ... for the children as well ... they always waiting for the husband to take them out they don't know how to go which way to go and how to follow maps and stuff and where to find these kind of places to go so it's more helpful for them as well that way.

> ... because you've got experienced mothers there, you always got somebody in different stages of pregnancy so you can come in and ask whatever you want about any stage of pregnancy or after, after you've had the baby, about the labour; you've got the midwives as well, you've got quite a variety of people to speak to and different issues you can bring up and a variety of experienced people you can ask so it's not just professional midwives; you can ask mothers because they've gone through the experience and you can have the experience of them as well, do you know what I mean?

A similar model has now been set up in a separate locality, with assistance from a Healthy Living Centre, again with local nursery accommodation.

Many of the women who have engaged with the projects wanted to work closely with the NHS to help women in their communities. Together with a health visitor colleague, the consultant midwife has facilitated the establishment of a health group for women in one locality. Maternity services will benefit as this forum provides the gateway to isolated non-English speaking communities. As the group also aims to enhance opportunity into NHS employment, this innovation supports the Trust's Ethnicity and Diversity Policy which aims to enhance the ethnic minority workforce in the NHS.

Some mothers have been trained as breastfeeding peer-supporters, working both in the hospital and the community, particularly in Sure Start groups. As part of their training, they have attended the two-day 'Baby Friendly' course devised for health professionals by the Infant Feeding Co-ordinator, a health visitor with Breastfeeding Network training, and one of the authors. This has provided invaluable insight for the health professionals into cultural issues, and the practical benefits of breastfeeding once the period of initiation, with which they are usually involved, has elapsed, and has generated frank feedback.

Other mothers, who have demonstrated a skill or a particular desire to stay in touch, were invited to take part in researching the issues of postnatal depression in their community. Their training as research workers has enabled the women to build their confidence, in addition to assisting their community with health information. Some have given presentations at conferences, and some are now becoming voluntary workers in the NHS.

Maternity services for ethnic minority women in Blackburn and Accrington are based on need, grounded in woman-centred philosophies and aim to build on women's strengths and beliefs rather than their risk factors. We strive to provide services in a non-patronising and non-judgmental way by being respectful, appropriate and kind. Through providing a culturally sensitive service, midwives have promoted a positive image, and have maximised both their own and women's personal potential.

REFERENCES

CEMD 2001 Confidential enquiry into maternal deaths. RCOG, London

Macpherson W (Chair) 1999 The Lawrence enquiry. Vols. 1 & 2 HMSO, London

ONS (Office for National Statistics) Mortality statistics in childhood,infant and perinatal for England and Wales Series. DH3 No 32

Payne J, Fleming A G 2002 Asian women's drop-in centre. MIDIRS Midwifery Digest 12(3):419-421

Richens Y 2003 Exploring the experiences of women of Pakistan origin of UK maternity services. DOH, London

Parent Education Classes for South Asian Women: Sampad

Editors

Two of the large maternity units in the West Midlands, with a multi-racial clientele, recognised that there was a problem in attracting women of South Asian origin to antenatal classes. While Asian Parentcraft courses were being run regularly, using link workers, attendance was generally very poor. The following issues were identified:

- the women were anxious about discussing intimate health matters with strangers
- some of the women spoke little or no English
- cultural taboos about the body inhibited the women from coming to classes
- the women often considered that senior female members of their families rather than health professionals were the appropriate people to give advice about pregnancy, birth and childcare. The maternity care system was therefore seen as unnecessary or inappropriate to help them prepare for birth.

Midwives with responsibility for parent education decided to collaborate with Sampad, an arts organisation dedicated to making music and creativity an important feature in the lives of children and their parents. The aim of the collaboration was to make antenatal health care as accessible as possible to the large numbers of women from a South Asian background who were not currently accessing services. It was hoped that this would be a positive step towards developing a relationship of trust between health professionals and Asian women, and would be helpful for health professionals in dispelling common stereotypes and misinformed beliefs about diverse cultural and religious values and practices.

Two days of intensive planning, involving the Sampad artists (a musician, trainee musician and two dancers) an active birth teacher, midwives and other hospital staff with responsibility for parent education, were undertaken.

Women were sent special invitations to attend the Sampad antenatal sessions. Publicity material indicated that the sessions would be informal, creative and entertaining. Hospital and clinic staff put up posters in local shops and community centres.

THE SESSIONS

Sampad aimed to ensure that the atmosphere at the sessions was relaxing and nurturing, and that the women felt safe and pampered. Community languages were used and sessions were Asian specific.

Staff provided refreshments for the women and dressed the room with saris. The inclusion of a social element at each session was critical. The time spent with a cup of tea and a biscuit allowed the women to talk to each other and to the midwives, and some of the less confident women had the chance to ask questions that they might not have been willing to put forward in a larger group.

PARTICIPANTS

Participants included Pakistani Muslim women, Punjabi Sikh women and Gujarati Hindus. Between 15 and 20 women attended each session. A significant proportion of the women were very young, some only 16 or 17 years old. They had recently come to Britain as brides, and were usually living with their husbands' parents. Some of the women arrived at the sessions in full burka, but soon disrobed when made to feel at home. They tended to be very shy and quiet, and spoke little or no English.

CONTENT of CLASSES

The Sampad artists and active birth teacher passed the leadership of the sessions seamlessly between them and adapted their material to respond to the needs of participants. Each session involved relaxation, massage, exercise, music and practical antenatal information.

Participatory singing centred on lullabies set to South Asian music, and an occasional English lullaby (several of the women said that their own mothers had sung 'Twinkle twinkle little star' to them). Care was taken to avoid Indian classical raags and folk songs which referred to Hindu gods as these would not have been acceptable to Muslim women. Instead, the musical content concentrated on songs common to a range of communities or on non-verbal singing. Relaxation visualisations to both live and recorded music were also included. As primary care-givers, the women taking part in the project were encouraged to look at music as a positive, creative part of everyday life.

Almost all of the women had never done any music before, so it was important to make them feel comfortable and to approach the singing very carefully. In the end, the singing was the aspect of the sessions that had the greatest emotional charge for both participants and observers. Some of the women were reduced to tears while singing lullabies that their mothers had sung to them, particularly as their mothers were often far away. Through the songs, the women made the connection between themselves as children and their impending motherhood, and deepened the bond with their unborn babies.

A Khathak dancer and a Bharatanatyam dancer demonstrated movements that could be useful in managing pain during labour, and taught breathing exercises for relaxation.

PARTICIPANT FEEDBACK

I really enjoyed everything especially the humming and singing and the massage.

I liked the music – it makes us relaxed.

I'm very glad I attended this class. I feel a lot more relaxed and confident about giving birth for the first time.

The lullabies were very nice to sing and relaxing.

It was very relaxing as I do not get much time at home to relax. I hope that they carry on having more sessions like the ones we have just had because I think a lot of women would find it very informative.

Encouraging Asian women to be involved is an excellent idea which will grow.

MIDWIFERY EVALUATION

The midwives felt that the project had been successful in:

- increasing the women's understanding of pregnancy and labour
- helping the women acquire skills for coping with labour, delivery and early parenting
- reducing stress and anxiety
- increasing knowledge of when professional help might be appropriate
- promoting community networking.

FUTURE DIRECTIONS

The project proved extremely successful in overcoming some of the barriers to class attendance which had originally been identified. Music making was used as a tool to reach a community that is often denied access both to creative expression and to informed choices in health care. Currently, the hospital principally involved in the project provides a rolling Asian Parentcraft programme of four week blocks. The suggestion now is to run the classes in blocks of five with the first session in each including music and dance and having a social emphasis. After this celebratory meeting which aims to draw the women in, subsequent sessions will cover the usual parentcraft information.

CONTACT DETAILS

Sampad South Asian Arts
c/o Midlands Arts Centre, Cannon Hill Park, Birmingham, B12 9QH
Tel: 0121 446 4312
Email: info@sampad.org.uk

The Albany Practice, South–East London: Antenatal and Postnatal Groups

Editors

The first antenatal group was set up in Deptford in the mid-1980s as a means of providing education, social contact, professional and peer support for local women. The group ran on a weekly basis as an informal session, with the women attending the group setting the agenda. Women could come to the group at any stage in their pregnancy, and for as many weeks as they wanted. Some women would come each week of their pregnancy from the moment they knew they were pregnant, and some would come every now and then. There was no need to advertise the group; women were encouraged to attend by their midwives, and other women heard about it through word of mouth. This continues to be the means of recruiting new members today.

After a while, some of the women said that they would like to bring their male partners. This was discussed and the women decided that they wanted to continue to have a women-only group and would like, therefore, to start another antenatal group which men could attend as well. Some of the women then came to both groups.

When women had given birth to their babies, they would come back to the antenatal group to talk about their experiences. This was fine until there were so many newborn babies and older babies present that the group became too big. At this point, it was decided to start a separate postnatal group. The women (and partners) would come back once to the antenatal group to show their babies and tell the others their birth stories, and would then move on to the postnatal group. Here they would meet many of the women they had known in the antenatal group, so that continuity of social contact was achieved.

All three groups continue to flourish today. There is no agenda for any of the sessions, although the women feel that the presence of the midwife as a facilitator is vital. Her job is to ensure that everyone has a chance to speak, and to provide information as and when needed. She ensures that women who are new to the group or who are lacking in confidence have a chance to speak. She is not seen by the group as the person with the answers; her role is to help people find solutions to their own problems by drawing on the experience of the other women. She is seen by the women as someone who recognises that there are lots of different solutions to problems and no one way of doing things. The women find this attitude empowering, and grow in confidence that they have the ability to make their own choices and the right decisions for their families.

Every session starts with introductions when each woman has the chance to talk about her week and anything that is worrying her. If there is something a woman wants to ask about, the group provides the space for her to do so. Issues are explored as deeply as the group wishes to take them. Not all the talk is about birth and babies. Other topics such as housing and maternity benefits frequently occur, and problems with partners are also discussed:

> It's allowed for you to have problems with your partner, whereas in other places, you're supposed to pretend that your relationship is perfect.

One of the most important aspects of the antenatal group is when women who have just given birth come back to talk about their labours, and their experiences of either home or hospital birth. This seems to help women learn in a far more powerful way than through formal instruction:

> It stayed in my head because the information was attached to a real person and was therefore absorbed differently.

Over the course of their pregnancies, the women hear about many different kinds of birth from women who come from very different backgrounds. They become very knowledgeable about labour as well as developing an understanding that each birth is unique. One woman commented that she felt she was receiving 'very rich information', and another said:

> The group covered everything because there were so many people coming through, you got a much wider set of experiences than if you'd gone to a class where they had set things each week.

The group functions at least as much as a support group as a group which people attend to gain information. Women who have attended the group say that it helped them to feel that they had the power to determine for themselves what they wanted to do:

> It made me more positive about every area because it's the sort of group that helps you go through everything and make your own decisions.

> It's not judgmental. You don't ever go away feeling that you're doing something wrong.

> You get confidence to do what you want to do.

Friendships develop on the basis of equality. Women attending the group, whether pregnant or new mothers, are seen as having their own expertise, and therefore as being in a position to share ideas and information with others.

The postnatal group provides the ongoing support the women need as they embark on the challenges of parenting. Women can attend the group for as long as they want, and enjoy watching the babies developing and growing up together. The atmosphere is not competitive:

It makes you feel OK about whatever your baby is doing.

These groups are a model of antenatal and postnatal education and support which could be replicated in many communities where women are isolated or lack confidence to attend traditional antenatal classes, or do not access services. The midwife is expected and welcomed in the group, but her role is principally to ensure that everyone feels included, to listen, and to encourage the group to find solutions to its own problems. The model is one of empowerment and support and its success can be seen in the fact that many of the women (and often partners as well) continue to meet for months or years afterwards, having established lasting friendships.

The Bellevue Project:
Local classes for local women

Editors

The aim of the Bellevue Project (Birmingham: May 2001 – September 2003) was to provide accessible, relevant maternity care to childbearing women in an area of high socio-economic need served by the Bellevue Medical Centre. A conventional model of team midwifery was replaced by a model of community midwifery fully integrated into the primary care setting. Parent education was a principal component of the enhanced service provided by a 0.7WTE midwife (Angela).

Angela ran one clinic per week at the Centre and this gave her the opportunity to get to know the local pregnant women well. Prior to the Project, women had had to travel to the hospital for parent education, a journey that involved taking two buses. Inevitably, most women did not go to classes. Angela set up her antenatal classes in a community flat next to the health centre, a comfortable and informal setting well known to the women.

Local classes run by a midwife already known to the women proved extremely successful with 92 women (63 primipara and 29 multipara) attending out of a total of 150 births during the two year period of the Project. A personal invitation to attend sessions was sent to each woman. Women were told that the classes would be a social event, that light refreshments would be offered and that their presence was eagerly sought because they would have so much to offer to the group. The women could attend at any stage of their pregnancy and come to as many or as few of the eight sessions as they wanted. There was no need to book.

Once they had attended one session, the women were generally keen to come to more. Quite often, they did not arrive at the beginning of a session or stay until the end. Angela put no pressure on the women to conform strictly to class times and this seemed to work well in terms of maintaining attendance.

The group attracted women's partners, siblings, friends, parents and grandparents as well as pregnant women from other areas. Approximately 64% of the pregnant participants were from minority ethnic groups. Many brought friends to interpret for them, and Angela developed her teaching to include a large proportion of visual aids. The group's understanding about birth and early parenting was often enhanced by women who had had their babies coming back to talk about their experiences.

Angela also set up a separate group for very young mothers, but this was not a success and the girls preferred to attend the mainstream sessions where they mixed very happily with the older women and indeed often took the lead. Teenage fathers also came along to some of the sessions to support their partners. All three women from the Bellevue practice list whose unborn babies were on the Child Protection 'At Risk' Register attended the groups. None of these women had received any parent education in their previous pregnancies.

A variety of other professionals worked alongside Angela at the parent education sessions. These included health visitors, sexual health outreach workers, a counsellor and student midwives. This enabled the women to establish a relationship with different health workers before the birth of their babies and ensured that they received a wide public health education. Yoga and baby massage sessions were also provided.

Key factors

Angela felt that the success of the parent education group depended on the following key factors:

- She coordinated all the classes
- The women invited to attend already knew her from the weekly clinic she ran at the Bellevue Practice
- Each woman was issued with a personal invitation to come to classes
- The classes were run at a local venue and were for local women
- They focused positively on normal labour and normal birth
- The diversity of parents attending enabled everyone to feel part of the group; no-one felt stigmatised or 'different'
- The group was family-focused and women were welcome to bring their children with them
- Women learned from the experiences of others who came back to the

group after having their babies
- The social aspect of the group was encouraged so that friendships were made and local support networks set up.

Evaluation

One hundred and thirty evaluation forms completed during the lifetime of the Project pointed to women's satisfaction with the parent education group.

Twenty-one women commented that they enjoyed *meeting other people, mums and babies.* They liked *people sharing their experiences and being able to ask questions.*

You don't get this opportunity during an antenatal appointment at the hospital.

They found the sessions *relaxing, enjoyable and reassuring* and would have liked *more time.*

Peer support and the chance to discuss worries and ask questions were highlighted as more important than information about pain relief in labour. Input during classes on breastfeeding was favourably commented upon and 83% of the women who completed the evaluation forms breastfed their babies.

Conclusion

The Report of the Bellevue Project (2003) concluded that:

Community based groups for the local population help to facilitate peer group support, as well as providing parent education including public health messages. This helps to focus on both short term and long term aims for the family. (p33)

Sadly, the funding for the Bellevue Project has come to an end and there is no longer a midwife dedicated to the Practice. Efforts are currently being made to find more funding and reinstate the parent education group.

Copies of the Report of the Bellevue Project are available from:
Perinatal Institute, St. Chad's Court, 2/3 Hagley Road, Birmingham B16 9RG
email: office@perinate.org
www.perinate.org/pc-aims

4U Teenage Pregnancy Group

Editors

Group leader: Lizzie

Started: November 2002

Target group: Girls must be under the age of 18 to attend the group

Funding: Lizzie is funded for 7.5 hours/week by the Teenage Pregnancy Partnership in Birmingham, and for 14.5 hours by the Solihull Teenage Pregnancy Partnership and a local NHS Trust.

Venue: Large teaching hospital – somewhat unexpectedly, a very popular venue. The young mothers like to meet in a place with which they are all familiar.

Recruiting clients: Lizzie works in the antenatal clinic where she tells teenage mothers about the group. Colleagues refer young mothers to her.

Advertising material: This has been designed specifically with young people in mind. Brightly coloured, glossy A5 flyers and A3 posters state:

U R invitd 2
4U

and ask:

R U Pregnant and under 18?

The sheet lists some of the topics that the group might discuss:

- Is there life after having a baby?
- Fashion while pregnant
- Breastfeeding
- Will it hurt?
- Can I get any money?
- What are my rights?
- What about my figure?
- College/School?

Business Cards in pink and blue washes advertise:
4U
Tuesdays 4 – 6.30p.m.
Parentcraft Room
Heartlands Hospital

Publicity: The group has been advertised on Radio 1, Heart FM, a Birmingham-based, popular music radio station, and on local TV.

Articles about the group have appeared in the local press.

Incentives: Food is provided at the start of every session. A small goodie bag with items for the baby and toiletries for the mother is given to every teenager who attends the group for 4 weeks.

Texting service: Lizzie uses a secure Internet site, accessed from a PC, to send out the same messages to everyone on the 4U list or individual messages. Clients are texted with reminders of the date of the next 4U meeting.

> **Hi welcome 2 yr 1st txt frm 4U teenage parentcraft grp. This is a grp this is definitely 4U. u can send a txt back as long as u do it within 2hrs of receivin this txt.**

Texts also convey brief health messages:

> **Hi hope u r enjoying sunshine. Hope 2 c u at 4U grp 2day at 4p.m. Doin relaxation so come & chill out. c u. Lizzie.**

> **Have a good valentines day! Did u know u can get free dental treatment while u r pregnant & 4 1 yr after baby born?**

Aims of the group:

- To build the young mothers' self-esteem
- To help them communicate effectively with health professionals
- To help them make friends with others in their own situation
- To provide a non-judgmental environment where they can freely express their thoughts and feelings
- To help them feel accepted

- To keep them in touch with services (antenatal checks are offered at the 4U sessions for teenagers who have not been attending clinic regularly, or who have specific concerns).

How the group runs: The agenda for the meeting is determined by the teenagers themselves, and the format is informal. The young mothers generally come with their boyfriend, mother, grandmother or a friend.

Visiting speakers:

- Dietician – who showed the teenagers how to make smoothies while talking to them about healthy diet in pregnancy
- Benefits advisor – because benefits are often a key issue for young mothers
- Young parents advisor – funded by the local Neighbourhood Renewal Fund
- Active birth teacher – who demonstrated massage techniques.

Young mothers who have previously attended the group come back with their babies and talk about their experiences. Health service planners also visit the group to consult the teenagers about the kind of services they want.

Videos: Videos are selected for their appeal to young people, e.g. extracts from *Friends* and *The Royle Family* have provided material for discussion about breastfeeding.

Future developments:

- A postnatal group (currently no funding available)
- A dads group (when a suitable father can be found to lead it)
- A dedicated antenatal clinic for teenage mums where they could talk to a midwife about anything that's worrying them while waiting for their check-up.

Feedback from mothers who have attended 4U:

I liked meeting other people who were pregnant and my age.

We could talk to each other cos we were going through the same things.

There was food and drink in case we were hungry.

We made a box to keep the baby stuff in.

I enjoyed it because I felt comfortable and reassured. Meeting other girls in my position helped me come to terms with my pregnancy.

What makes the group so successful?

- Sticking rigidly to the under 18-rule. Very young mothers will not attend a group which includes 18 and 19 year olds and older teenagers have very different needs from younger ones.
- The fact that the person leading the group is totally committed to young parents and is enthusiastic about the work she is doing. Young people are very sensitive to any lack of interest or hostility on the part of carers.

Blackburn Teenage Mothers' Group

Clare Harding

Queen's Park Hospital Maternity Unit serves a varied and culturally diverse population in Blackburn. Of the annual 3,500 births, 366 babies last year were born to 'teenage' mothers. Immediately this phrase is used, assumptions crowd in. Some of these babies were dearly wanted, others were unplanned. Some of their mothers were in stable relationships, others were single; some had their own accommodation, some were homeless, others lived at home with their parents; some had literacy problems, others had, or went on to gain, a string of educational qualifications; some had good role models, others, poor or absent role models; some had good support, others needed to find great reserves of strength and courage to cope alone. All these statements equally apply to mothers from any age group. Some young women in their teens have a greater ability to parent than others in their twenties or thirties, others find it hard to meet their own needs, let alone those of another demanding human being (Hudson, 2002).

Obstetrically, young mothers are at no greater risk than the rest of the child-bearing population, and have a significantly lower caesarean rate (Edwards, 2000). They may arguably be able to cope better than their older counterparts with the lack of sleep and the changing life-style a baby brings. However, many young mothers have to deal with poverty and prejudice. In public health, the emphasis is on reducing teenage pregnancy, little use to those who already pregnant (SEU, 1999; Chambers et al, 2001). It is against this background that we need to examine young mothers' education for birth and parenthood.

Rozette et al (2000) found that the pregnant schoolgirls they interviewed described health professionals, for example, as *judgmental, patronising, and felt that they treated young mothers differently*. Ninety-five per cent of them would have liked young mother discussion groups. The sensitivity of these mothers makes it easy for them to feel discrimination. In addition, some have already had negative experiences of schooling. Their education needs – information, communication and choice – are the same as those of any other mother. It is its delivery which needs to reflect a mutual respect, improve self-esteem, be interactive, and, above all, be fun.

School-age mothers in Blackburn attend a special unit, St. Thomas's, where parent education, given by a midwife, forms a part of the curriculum. A second midwife was recruited to work with young mothers, and to develop a drop-in group. A young woman who had become a mother at 16 was also identified to train as a Teenage Pregnancy Support Worker, to liaise with teenagers, and encourage them to attend (Quinn & Harding, 2001). Both midwives attended a six-day ENB approved workshop on facilitating antenatal education. This addressed the midwives' needs for facilitation skills, and modelled client-centred approaches with practical experience of interactive techniques and small group work, which not only stimulate discussion and promote learning, but also help to build up peer support (Nolan, 1998; Schott & Priest, 2002). It is vital to consider the literacy levels of the mothers, but that does not mean making assumptions, or 'watering down'. The best education starts with what the student already knows, and by working in small groups, the more literate help the less.

The peer worker attended a 20-hour course on running groups, which identified her strengths and learning needs. It covered practical aspects, cultural issues, listening and communication skills and group-work. It was followed by 10 hours' supervision, in which problems and questions could be discussed, and the work audited. This mother went out on the streets, meeting teenagers and discovering their needs. The young mothers' group was launched at an open day held at the local College of Further Education. One consideration in choosing venues has been proximity to education, as one of the aims of the support work is to encourage return to education after the birth. Another is the availability of crèche facilities. This day was full of activities for the young parents, rather than being simply focused on the baby. Food and pampering have always proved powerful incentives, and are still important elements. The weekly group has continued, with mothers from St. Thomas's joining in, despite this extending their school day (Cheema, 2002).

The peer worker found that helping the mothers negotiate the housing and benefits systems and helping with reading were as important as discussing parenting. She helped the group to plan trips out, as many had never been out of their immediate locality. Improving her own literacy and IT skills, she and the group designed a booklet giving local information and options for pregnant young women, the information that she would have liked at the age of 15. This is now in its second edition (Cunliffe, 2001). The peer worker gained tremendously in confidence, as she addressed groups of health workers, and mastered Powerpoint in order to speak and give a presentation at a Royal College of Midwives conference.

A male midwife (who also attended the six-day course) ran a group for young fathers which met over the lunch they prepared themselves. Again, the emphasis was on practical skills, valuing and respect; on modelling rather than telling.

Many examples demonstrate the building of self-esteem fostered by the group, such as the training of teenage mothers from Sure Start areas to act as breastfeeding peer-supporters. They have attended the two-day 'Baby Friendly' course devised for health professionals by the Infant Feeding Co-ordinator, a health visitor with Breastfeeding Network training, and the author. This has provided invaluable insight for participating health professionals, has challenged stereotypes and has generated frank feedback. During the 2003 Breastfeeding Awareness Week, a photograph of three young breastfeeding mothers was used locally in promoting breastfeeding amongst teenage mothers. It is now used, with their permission, on the cover of breastfeeding information given to *all* mothers Mothers have designed publicity material, and have given presentations to midwives and at conferences, such as the recent Teenage Pregnancy Unit Joint Royal College of Midwives and Department of Health Policy Forum.

One sometimes meets educators who complain that 'their teenagers' won't participate. All expectant parents have anxieties about classes, and letting them know what to expect, and that the sessions will meet their needs rather than tell them what to do, is vital. I remember the 19 year-old mother who berated her peers for smoking after giving birth to a small baby, the young woman who confided that she wasn't going to do anything in the group, but who became the scribe feeding back from the very first small group work, the young man who said he didn't write who organised his group to label the birth atlas, and the father who got his group to try out the positions he and his partner had found useful. At the end of the session, this father said:

I'd be a birth supporter for any woman in this room (there were nearly 50!) It was brilliant. It was the best day of my life.

REFERENCES

Chambers R, Wakley G, Chambers S 2001 Tackling teenage pregnancy. Radcliffe Medical Press, Abingdon

Cheema K 2002 Supporting pregnant teenagers. MIDIRS 12(1):26-29

Cunliffe L 2001 Information for pregnant young women under 25. BHRV Health Care Trust, Blackburn

Edwards G 2000 Teenage pregnancies: comparative outcomes. Practising Midwife 3(6):12-15

Hudson F 2002 Supporting young parents. In: Nolan M (ed) Education and support for parenting. Ballière Tindall, Edinburgh

Nolan M 1998 Antenatal education: a dynamic approach. Ballière Tindall, Edinburgh

Quinn P, Harding C 2001 Involving clients and responding to women's needs. Midwives in Action: a resource. English National Board, London

Rozette C, Houghton-Clemmey R, Sullivan K 2000 A profile of teenage pregnancy: young women's perceptions of the maternity services. Practising Midwife 3(10):23-25

Schott J, Priest J 2002 Leading antenatal classes: a practical guide. Books for Midwives, Oxford

SEU (Social Exclusion Unit) 1999 Teenage pregnancy. HMSO, London

The Café Class (National Childbirth Trust)

Alexandra Smith

At home I refer to the two hours I spend drinking coffee on Monday mornings as my Café Class. I use the term deliberately in order to stress to my family and others that I am working despite appearances to the contrary. With the women I drink coffee with, I avoid the word 'class' deliberately, the principle being that, in a setting such as a café, learning is an organic and fluid process with personal growth happening naturally and easily. In a classroom setting, however flexible and well informed the teaching approach, learning is often inhibited by externally or internally imposed restraints or expectations. The traditional antenatal class is often an 'artificial' event because it is separate from any other aspect of a person's life. People learn best when they are relaxed and free from anxiety – but a class that asks people to write and speak in front of others, or take part in an unfamiliar group exercise will inevitably trigger some degree of apprehension. Only a minority of adults really enjoy the challenge of this kind of learning environment. On the other hand, the majority of people are very comfortable meeting friends in the café – especially if they don't know it's really a class.

I started the café meetings about eighteen months ago because of my beliefs about education and also because of the geographical nature of rural Wales. Women approaching the National Childbirth Trust, for which I work, at any one time are likely to live over a wide area and be at very different stages of pregnancy. Many would find it hard to commit to a conventional course of NCT classes for financial reasons as well as difficulties with transport. Often women contact me because they are new to the area and want to make friends.

My general aims are for participants:

- To become aware of their needs and know how these can be met
- To become part of a 'community of birthing women'
- To benefit from peer group support and learning
- To develop insight into a range of childbirth and parenting issues
- To develop self confidence and self esteem as women and parents.

Women are welcome at any stage of pregnancy or early parenting. The café provides a central and easily accessible meeting point where people can come together as part of their morning in town. I arrive at 10.00am with *The Guardian* crossword (in case it is a quiet morning) and stay until 12.00. There may be just one or two people one week and up to seven another. The group continues to meet on the Mondays I cannot attend and recently some of the members with crawling and toddling babies have started an afternoon meeting in a more suitable venue. Some people come for the whole two hours, and others for a shorter time. Fathers (and grandmothers) occasionally 'call in' for a few minutes to say hello – but essentially it is a women's forum. I run additional sessions at home for women approaching the birth. Partners come to these sessions as well and we share a meal together.

I feel my role is to:

- Introduce newcomers into the group
- Establish the specific needs of each individual
- Facilitate discussion and learning when appropriate
- Listen, affirm and show respect – thus establishing the 'tone' of the group

- Hold babies, on request.

Learning takes place almost entirely through discussion, though practical skills such as nappy folding, putting a baby sling on, and holding a baby are passed on quite naturally within the group – and the visual impact of seeing babies breastfed and cared for in a social setting is very powerful. The informal and relaxed setting leads to a natural flow of discussion that is rather different from the more focused or formal discussion that might occur in a class setting. Being group led, the discussion is always specific to the immediate needs of an individual and there is a very high level of intergroup exchange.

Topics frequently discussed include:

- Maternity care choices and antenatal testing
- Place of delivery
- How the system works – and working the system
- Communicating with health professionals
- Research-based evidence
- All aspects of pregnancy
- Different birth experiences – physical and emotional
- Practical advice on arranging water birth
- The impact of early parenting
- Sleeping arrangements with a new baby
- Breastfeeding
- Baby equipment and baby care
- Immunisation and Vitamin K
- Relationships
- Returning to work/study.

Returning to the need I have to consider myself to be working, what do I actually do? I have had to analyse this in order to justify the simplicity of this approach to learning and the apparent lack of structure. I do still use a wide range of facilitation and teaching skills but these appear to be entirely hidden – my verbal input is often minimal. One of our members said recently, 'It struck me that I'd never thought of the meetings in the cafe as "teaching" or as "education" in any way.' I think members regard me as a friend/older sister/mother figure – but I am aware that I use counselling skills to underpin the group dynamic and establish the ethos of the group and this will make the group different from an entirely 'un-led' one.

Counselling skills include:

- Developing and showing empathy
- Being open myself – genuineness
- Showing warmth and acceptance – unconditional positive regard (or respect)

- Building trust and confidence within the group – confidentiality
- Active listening
- Interpersonal skills.

Women don't need antenatal classes to be able to give birth and parent – but they do need opportunities to gather, discuss and assimilate information if they are to make informed decisions about the things other people want to do to them and their babies.

Learning outcomes for the café meetings are difficult to set or measure, as there is no specific agenda for these sessions. Evaluation to date has been by informal observation of contributory behaviour, continuing attendance, verbal feedback, sustained friendships and, importantly, the changes that people make as a direct consequence of participation. Based on this I believe the approach has been successful – though the numbers involved are very small.

Chapter 8

Education for Birth and Parenting: where next?

Mary Nolan

Government wants family-centred maternity services that are accessible to all sections of the childbearing community. It also wants services that are cost-effective. Research shows quite clearly that there is a close link between maternal mental health and the wellbeing of infants. The influence of the early involvement of fathers in family life in terms of enhancing children's life experiences is now recognised. Education for birth and parenting has a significant part to play in fulfilling every aspect of the government and research agenda for families. It can increase women's awareness of their own resources for coping with labour and thereby reduce demands for costly interventions such as epidurals and caesarean section. It can also help women prepare for the stresses of early motherhood and provide them with a peer group to support them. It can show men what role they can play in birth and early parenting, and explain just how important that role is. Responsible, highly trained childbirth educators are not a luxury in today's cost-conscious and consumer-orientated maternity care services; they are essential.

(Editors' note)

Those involved in running groups for expectant parents, or in working with individual women, individual couples or families, will be very aware that pregnancy is a unique and precious moment for education. Even adults who left school some years previously, disillusioned with the process of learning, will present themselves at antenatal classes, prepared to give education another 'go' in the interests of getting ready for the birth of their baby and adjusting to new responsibilities. Adults with extremely demanding jobs will come to classes straight from work, carrying briefcases and wearing formal clothes. A recent class of mine included a woman whose life had been crippled by myalgic encephalomyelitis (ME) for several years. By evening, she was invariably exhausted and she and her partner rarely went out.

Nevertheless, she came to every class in the five-week series and participated in all the physical activities we undertook, even if she sometimes had to do them sitting down. On the same Lichfield course was another woman who arrived at one class, breathless, just in time for the 7p.m. start, having been at a meeting in Dusseldorf at 7.30 in the morning, and attended another meeting in London in the middle of the day. The social mix in this particular group included people working as security guards, teachers, financiers, secretaries, lorry drivers, nurses and one unemployed person. At the end of the final class, we did a carousel exercise where people sat facing each other in two circles and spent three minutes talking to the person opposite them about a variety of parenting topics before moving on to talk to another person about another topic. I asked them to discuss the following:

- Why is being a father so hard today?
- What will be the most difficult thing about the first week at home with your baby? How will you cope?
- What would it be like to be a mother who chooses to stay at home to look after her baby? What would it be like to go back to work?
- Which of your relationships is going to be most difficult to manage after the birth of your baby?
- How would you cope if your child turned out to be exceptionally talented? How would you cope if your child turned out to be less intelligent than you anticipate?
- What two things have struck you most about this course?

The enormous swell of conversation which followed as soon as each new topic was handed out testified to the fact that the 18 people who had attended the course had found a commonality of interests that might not perhaps have been predicted on the basis of their socio-economic backgrounds.

Muller-Staffelstein (1996) comments on the exceptional window of opportunity provided by pregnancy:

> The group parents-to-be (as compared to the average adult) shows an above-average openness and is easily motivated to learn and to reflect on old roles and habits; for example, their relationship to their own bodies, to pleasure and pain, to body signals, to their use of medications. The process of pregnancy also stimulates examining one's positions concerning autonomy, independence, security, risk and responsibility, control and trust, and perhaps to reposition. (p75)

As previous chapters in this book have so clearly demonstrated, teaching in pregnancy should be richly textured to assist cognitive, affective and social learning. The parents-to-be set their own agenda. The educator's role is then to facilitate detailed exploration of this agenda in order to develop parents' understanding of their own needs and capacity to make decisions that are right for them. In addition, the educator hopes through her skilful delivery of classes or running of groups to impact on parents' feelings about and attitudes towards education, stimulating a reassessment of its place in their own lives and of what its place in their child's life might be.

The value that parents-to-be place on antenatal education will most certainly be influenced by the value which educators and the institutions which the educators represent are seen to place on it. A colleague recently appointed as Parent Education Coordinator at a large teaching hospital in the Midlands came into post to discover that there was no budget allocated to her, that she had no office, no computer and no telephone, and that there was no room at the hospital dedicated to parent education. For the first two years, she taught classes wherever she could find the space – in the hospital canteen, in the antenatal clinic waiting area, in the outpatients reception and on one occasion, on a ward that had been temporarily closed. Such makeshift arrangements sent out the strongest of messages to parents that the hospital placed very little value on preparation for birth and parenting. With a caesarean section rate of 30% during these same two years, most of my friends' clients probably came to the conclusion that the hospital was far more committed to technology than to education!

Adults will not value learning that is obviously not valued by the person or the institution delivering it. Writing about ten parentcraft classes she observed, Underdown (1998) noted that eight of the ten started late, yet the clients *seemed to accept this unquestioningly*. In her paper, she speculates whether this *lack of irritation at the late start could have been due to low expectations* (p66), a poor starting point for learning. Clients will also make assumptions based on the environment in which classes are provided. If the room is clearly unsuited to physical skills work – to trying out different comfort positions for labour, to practising massage and relaxation techniques – then parents will quite logically conclude that these elements of the course are not particularly important. If there are no facilities for making a drink and no biscuits provided, parents will assume that classes are not supposed to be a social occasion where they are meant to enjoy talking to each other and exchanging experiences. If the visual aids used by the educator are tatty, out of date and unattractive, parents will assume that antenatal classes have passed their sell-by date, with no one committed to producing new and relevant visual aids for educators to use.

If the classes start late, the educator is unprepared, the teaching aids are poor, the chairs are hard and no refreshments are provided – yet the hospital or clinic has a brand new reception area, brand new fetal electronic monitoring equipment, and the patients' newspaper talks proudly of the number of operations being performed – is it surprising that pragmatic adult learners decide their time is wasted with the childbirth educator?

At a time when health professionals and the public alike are becoming increasingly aware that resources are finite, and that they must be paid for out of the country's hard-earned money, it is madness to waste an educational opportunity which 50% of first time parents in the UK wish to take up (Hancock, 1994); in Australia, it is 84% (Rolls & Cutts, 2001). With government giving strong support to primary prevention programmes, education for birth and parenting should surely now have its day. A pregnancy-long programme of classes, or better still, a pre-pregnancy to post-pregnancy programme, could make a significant contribution to improving the health and lifestyles of mothers and, through them, of their families. If obesity and depression are the diseases currently scourging western societies, education during pregnancy provides a wonderful opportunity to help people understand the roots of such ill health and the means of preventing it. Women and their partners can be persuaded to make drastic lifestyle changes in the interests of their babies when they would not make them in their own interests.

If antenatal education is to become a key component of a coherent primary prevention programme in the UK, it needs to restructure itself to provide education that is family, parenting and lifestyle centred (with birth seen as the catalyst for individual and social growth). It can no longer focus exclusively on labour, proselytise to promote conformity to medical protocols and ignore women's personal and social circumstances. This does not mean that education for birth is not important. Far from it – education for birth becomes the lynchpin of a strategy to enhance women's confidence in and respect for their own bodies; to strengthen the shared responsibilities of families and health professionals for achieving and maintaining physical health and mental wellbeing, and to increase understanding of the interface between nature and technology. However, any tendency to evaluate antenatal education solely in terms of the events which occur in the delivery room must be resisted. As Muller-Staffelstein (1996) explains, we need to redefine education for birth and parenting so that its perspectives are far broader and its effectiveness is judged on long-term outcomes:

> *Its meaning (pregnancy support and childbirth preparation) results from the support of the mother-to-be and her child, at the same time influencing the future developments of the child through primary prevention, thus giving further health-encouraging impulses. (p77)*

We know sufficient about the link between maternal mental health and children's wellbeing (Brockington, 1996) to be able to make a very strong case for education for birth and parenting as a primary prevention measure. The months of pregnancy can be dedicated to raising the self-confidence and self-esteem of parents-to-be. This is certainly not the time to persuade them by every means possible that a woman's body is ill-equipped to nurture a growing baby, and anatomically and physiologically unsuited to giving birth. It is not the time to persuade couples that they should delegate decision making about birth and early parenting to others. This is the time to educate adults for a richer adulthood, based on greater awareness of their own values in life, of the influences which affect their thinking, and increased confidence in their ability to make their own choices. Education for birth and parenting is essentially education for adulthood:

> Education functions as ... the 'practice of freedom', the means by which men and women deal critically and creatively with reality and discover how to participate in the transformation of their world. (Shaull, 1972)

Advice on diet, smoking, alcohol, drugs and sexual practices is rarely, if ever, welcomed by adults. When given, there is no guarantee that it will be acted upon. Indeed, health promotion campaigns telling people *not* to do certain things invariably fail – witness the increase in the numbers of young people, and especially young women, taking up smoking despite aggressive government warnings of the link between cigarettes and fatal diseases. Skilled educators leading early pregnancy classes help parents share their knowledge about healthy lifestyles, reach their own conclusions and make their own decisions in the context of their unique personal, domestic and social circumstances. Only the changes which are the result of adults making their own choices are likely to be long-lasting. Antenatal education has to replace advice with relevant information, and support for parents to make and enact decisions. This, as Wickham and Davies have illustrated in Chapter 5, requires health professionals to abandon the role of experts and become facilitators.

Antenatal classes provide an ideal opportunity to help women and men form a support network to assist them through and beyond the transition to parenthood. Schneider's study (2001) shows, as others have done (e.g. Jansen & Blizzard, 1999; Nolan, unpublished work, 1999), that women came to classes to meet other people in a similar situation Of the 13 women who attended the index course, 12 spoke warmly about their particular group and intended to keep in touch with at least one other person, and often several. Whether the group becomes a support group, and how vigorously the group functions, depends on the commitment of the educator to helping parents get to know each other, respect each other's views, listen to each other's ideas, and learn from each other. This will be achieved in large part through the respect the educator herself accords to each individual, and whether the process of her teaching sends out strong messages to the parents-to-be that:

- Your ideas are important and worth listening to.
- You can make your own decisions.
- Your decisions may be different from those made by other people, because your life circumstances are different from everyone else's.
- You have the ability to give birth to your child and to parent your child.
- What you know and the experiences you have had can help other people as their knowledge and experiences can help you.

What would family-centred education for birth and parenting look like? We don't have to start from scratch if we want to design a totally new kind of programme for parents in the UK. Firstly, there are plenty of pockets of good practice up and down our own country where community-based education, sometimes for very vulnerable and needy groups, is already in place. Examples of these are given in Chapter 7. We can also look to the international literature for guidance. Haskins Westmoreland and Zwelling (2000:31) describe the topics covered during their integrated pre-conception/antenatal/postnatal educational package:

- Pre-conceptual health course: *Can We? Should We?*
- Early pregnancy class: *Now We've Done It!*
- Mid-pregnancy course: *Decisions, Decisions, Decisions*
- Last trimester preparation for birth: *Here We Go!*
- Breastfeeding course: *So That's What They're For!*
- Postpartum support group for mothers: *Mom's Connection*
- Newborn course: newborn care and behaviour: *What Do We Do With Her Now?*
- Newborn course: *Intellectual and Emotional Care of the Newborn*
- Parenting course: *Parental Adjustments*
- Parenting course: *Boot Camp for Dads*

This is a demanding programme, setting very high standards for educational encounters that are considered to be of vital significance to parents-to-be and new parents. Haskins Westmoreland and Zwelling (2000) discuss how important it is for the long-term emotional significance of the childbearing experience to be addressed throughout their series of courses. This means that educators must understand its significance in their own lives before they can help others to appreciate its significance in theirs. A commitment to birth, and an understanding of the many and varied ways in which women and their families experience it, is therefore an essential prerequisite.

Also critical to the success of these educators' courses is, first and foremost, limiting the number of individual women or couples who attend. An ideal number is considered to be between 6 and 10 couples or 12 to 20 people. With larger groups, the social aspect of the course – getting to know other parents-to-be and networking with them – and the quality of the learning that can take place are diminished. Where people are intimidated by large numbers, they are unwilling to share and less able to listen well so that learning in the affective domain does not happen. It is difficult for the teacher to build the confidence of people whom she does not know as individuals.

The programme run by Haskins Westmoreland and Zwelling (2000) includes:

> Discussion of consumer rights and responsibilities for making informed choices based on knowledge of alternatives [with] the thread of informed choice ... woven throughout the entire curriculum. (p32)

In order to be able to provide unbiased information for parents-to-be and promote discussion which allows them freedom to formulate their ideas and apply them within their own life situations, teachers must be aware of their own standpoints on the management of birth and parenting styles. Such insight into where one is 'coming from' requires time spent in structured reflection on key experiences where choices were made or denied.

The penultimate criterion for success in the Haskins Westmoreland and Zwelling (2000) programme is:

> Family input and evaluation of class content and processs ... actively sought and used to improve classes. (p33)

This means ongoing consultation with parents-to-be as they go through the programme and, even more importantly, consultation with them after their babies are born and some months later with a view to establishing how the programme could be improved to make it more relevant to the 'real' experience of birth and early parenting. Nolan's research (1999) demonstrates clearly that parents of infants a few months old are well placed to define the contemporary parenting agenda and keep educators up-to-date when their own children may be well past infancy. One hundred and sixty-eight men and women attending NHS and NCT antenatal classes were asked before starting their classes, immediately after they had completed classes, and a couple of months after the birth of their babies, what they felt were the most important topics that should be covered in classes:

> The largest category of responses at each stage of questionnaire completion was that which subsumed all the postnatal topics requested by the subjects. This category was further analysed and broken down

into subsections of 'babycare skills' and 'life-changes after the birth'. By far the larger sub-section was that concerned with 'babycare skills' and typical responses are listed below:

'general advice on how to care for a new baby in the early days at home' (woman attending NHS classes: pre-classes questionnaire)

'recommended lotions, ointments, nappies etc.'
(father attending NCT classes: post-classes questionnaire)

(Nolan, 1999:160-161)

After their babies had been born, they were able to fine tune this agenda and provide a very detailed account of what they now understood their needs to have been.

'parentcraft: how to bathe the baby, safety in the home etc.' (woman attending NCT classes: post-birth questionnaire)

'common changes in babies e.g. cradle cap, milk spots, wind, colic etc. More information about this kind of thing – bathing and how often' (father attending NHS classes: post-birth questionnaire)

(Nolan, 1999:161)

Such evaluation cannot be done once and for all as the learning needs of parents will change as the society in which they live changes. Educators cannot assume that the parenting agenda for 1999 is relevant to the parents-to-be of 2004.

Finally, Haskins Westmoreland and Zwelling (2000) insist that childbirth educators must be certified, that is, they must have a qualification specifically in education for birth and parenting. These researchers warn against assuming that a qualification as a health professional implies possession of the skills required to be an effective educator. As teachers must *utilise a variety of teaching strategies during each class to meet the needs of different types of learners* (p32), they need a firm understanding of how humans learn, and of adult learning in particular. The training of teachers has to incorporate both educational theory and experimentation with teaching strategies to enable adults to learn effectively whatever their prefered learning style. Practice should first be undertaken with peers in the environment of the training institution, and later, with parents-to-be under the supervision of an experienced teacher. Constructive feedback on teaching, using the evaluation cycle to enable improvements to be made in future classes, is essential. Without the feedback of a trained observer, teachers must rely on the feedback given by parents which is useful but may be limited, either because clients have difficulty expressing exactly what they feel about classes, or because they are unwilling to criticise the teacher; and on their own assessment of their performance which may also be limited if they are new to the field of education for birth and parenting. In order to retain the status of certified educator, teachers must attend ongoing training events and provide evidence that they are keeping up-to-date. Lothian (2001) talks of the *veritable explosion of research related to pregnancy, birth and breastfeeding* and asserts that childbirth educators therefore *have a responsibility to seek out new knowledge and incorporate that knowledge into their practice.* (pix)

It is, of course, going to be extremely difficult to implement such an extensive and demanding programme of courses for birth and early parenting in a culture where such education is seen as a 'Cinderella' service which can safely be under-resourced or not resourced at all, and provided or not provided at the will of managers and health service accountants. However, it may be that the auditors and the accountants can be appeased. If women and their families have a positive experience of birth and the early weeks of parenting because of the education they received from midwives in the antenatal period and the ongoing support provided by their learning group in the postnatal period, they will be more likely to return to the hospital where the midwives work for their second and subsequent births, and indeed for other health services that they need during their lives. This makes it more likely that Primary Care Trusts will purchase services from these hospitals.

A vigorous programme of antenatal and postnatal education, wherever it is provided, targets young working people who have a strong voice in their communities, who will be using nurseries, child care facilities and schools; people who have contact with many other young parents and will influence them about what kind of health care they should seek and where. This will impact on the services provided at primary care level. Parents who have attended the GP surgery for weekly or monthly classes from early pregnancy until their babies are six months old, and have enjoyed both the educational and social aspects of their classes, are likely to view the practice favourably and will market it without any effort on the part of managers!

There are also long-term savings to be made when the family unit is strong and well-informed. Bryan (2000) claims that *interventions that increase mutual support in the couple unit can provide an important cost-effective method for facilitating family health* (p144). Bringing up children is probably the most stressful task that we undertake during our lives, and parenting is the area in which we are most vulnerable and require most support. This applies to all parents-to-be, whatever their circumstances. Campion (1997) describes how teaching parents with cognitive disabilities how to stimulate their children appropriately so that they can reach their full potential needs to be underpinned by *a lot of attention, support and caring ... given to the <u>parent</u>* (p13). The creation of a peer group during antenatal classes, whose members will be facing the various challenges presented by growing children at the same time, is a most powerful means of assisting women and men to tackle those challenges successfully. Antenatal education which continues into the postnatal period, when the emphasis on education may change gradually into an emphasis on mutual support, can play its part in nurturing healthy children through supporting their parents.

We disregard the mother's and the family's need for support at the peril of the wellbeing of the next generation. It is possible that there has never been a time when parents have been more in need of support. The complexities of modern living, the multiplicity of choices to be made in every area of life, and the speed of social, economic and political change make it essential that they receive support and become lifelong learners in the interests of raising children able to adapt successfully to a society where it is the norm for tomorrow to be a world entirely different from today. Maushart (1997) comments that *parents do not cope instinctively but by having developed a complex matrix of social learning, networks and support systems, and that when these systems have not existed or break down or falter ... the coping as a parent can be all the more difficult* (p101).

The link between maternal mental health and the long-term emotional and physical health of the child is now well established (Caplan et al, 1989; Barlow et al, 2002). The person most likely to support the mother in the critical early months of the new baby's life is her partner. Thus, in order to assist the mother to remain confident in herself and happy with her new status as mother, we need to have educated fathers who are able to offer practical help with caring for the baby, and emotional support because they have had the opportunity to anticipate and plan for the hurdles which must be surmounted by couples becoming parents.

Antenatal classes provide an opportunity for partners to gain a better understanding of their relationship with each other. The women attending the classes studied by Schneider (2001) spoke of the opportunity the antenatal course gave them to *share time with their partner* (p15). Childbirth and parenting educators can encourage couples to reflect together on information given, and to discuss how they can incorporate what they have learned into their plans for the birth and their lives afterwards. Work on the couple's relationship during the antenatal period may provide a buffer against the well documented stresses of the first three months of a baby's life when many new parents experience a decline in relationship satisfaction (Ross, 2001:562).

Men attending antenatal classes have reported being ignored or made to feel that they are not integral to the birth and early months of their baby's life. Their needs and feelings are not considered, but only what they can do to help their partners. They feel unprepared for the emotional aspects of parenting, and are very rarely helped to acquire the basic babycare skills which would allow them to participate more fully in the early postnatal weeks (Smith, 1999). As Beardshaw and Burgess have pointed out (Chapter 4), involving men fully in antenatal education may be the most effective means of easing the mother's transition to motherhood, and supporting the strength and quality of the couple's relationship during the early challenging months of their baby's life. Schmied et al (2002) provide evidence from Sydney that men who attend classes based on adult education principles and where gender-specific discussion groups are used, experience increased satisfaction with their early parenting experiences.

Current government rhetoric stresses the importance of consumers of health care being able to make informed choices. The concept of informed choice is flawed in so far as it is impossible to define exactly what being informed means. If we accept that no one can ever be fully informed, we are forced to define informed as sufficiently informed. Who decides when the consumer is sufficiently informed? The health professional or the consumer? If the health professional, does this not reinforce the traditional patriarchy of the health service – I will decide how much it is good for you to know; there are some things it is best if only I know? If the consumer, how do we prevent people from opting out of knowing, from abandoning decision-making and leaving it up to professionals who can then be conveniently blamed if anything goes wrong?

Leaving aside the fact that too close a scrutiny of the concept of informed choice is likely to result in its disintegration, let us accept that it is useful in terms of attempting to shift the balance of power away from health professionals and towards consumers. The concept is underpinned by a vision of the informed consumer of health-care services, actively participating in health-care decisions, synthesising professional knowledge with their unique understanding of their personal circumstances, and making choices for which they accept responsibility.

At present, both health professionals and the general public are a long way from realising such a mature approach to health care. Antenatal education for birth and parenting may be a starting point in the maturation process. It can help service users understand how to obtain the information they need from health professionals, how to weigh the evidence in relation to their own unique understanding of their physical and mental health needs, how to communicate their decisions to carers, and how to manage the outcomes of those decisions. Wilkerson (2000) argues that in adult education, *there should be an emphasis on developing intellectual capabilities such as analytic, problem-solving and critical-thinking skills* (p16). The aim is to increase responsibility, not to take it away, to increase the capacity for independence, not to diminish it. This can be achieved when the childbirth and parenting educator sees her role as, and is skilled in being:

- *a designer of ways to engage expectant parents in thoughtful problem-solving and decision-making*
- *a developer of questions that inspire reading, observation, analysis and reflection upon desired care and outcomes during the learners' birthing experiences*
- *a nurturer of curiosity, the creative drive and the search for a satisfying birth experience*
- *a nurturer of assertiveness. (Wilkerson, 2000:16)*

This is in keeping with the inspirational work of Paulo Freire (1972) who defined a pedagogy for the oppressed. Freire's notion of freeing the people through education, teaching them to analyse social and political structures, and to define and fight for their own role in local and national power structures aimed to liberate the oppressed peasants of South America. The breadth and courage of his thinking should not deter us from applying it to the Western world where the education of the people would lead to desired changes in the delivery of services. Those who mistrust the wisdom of users of services should remember that people will rarely ask for something that a rational assessment of the pros and cons shows would not benefit them or might harm them. If they do, the reason why must be strong enough to warrant investigation. It seems extremely likely that an informed mass of childbearing families would have a major impact on maternity services, starting with a significant reduction in the caesarean section rate. Sagady (2001) defines the preventable caesarean section and the role which childbirth educators can play in helping parents-to-be understand that:

> *A preventable cesarean is one which, while medically justified at the time of the actual procedure, may have been potentially prevented earlier in the labor by initiating certain interventions (or abstaining from others) which could influence the factors that ultimately led to the need for the cesarean (p30).*

Some may argue that parents-to-be do not want increased responsibility for their own care and that of their baby, that they are too frightened to choose autonomy rather than dependence. Little research has been done in this area, but the Ontario study by Sims-Jones et al, (1999) of 506 women and men attending prenatal classes found that 79.8% of clients starting classes were interested in a topic entitled 'dealing with your doctor', and that many of these felt that not enough time had been spent on this topic by the end of the prenatal course.

Empowering childbirth education could be the driving force behind a new – or rediscovered – understanding of birth that allows women to be in charge of their labour because it is accepted that they can birth their babies without costly, time-consuming and demeaning medical interventions. Today women cannot learn about childbirth informally through seeing other women give birth and supporting them during labour, because birth is no longer a domestic and community event; it is an event which takes place in an environment with which the woman is unfamiliar. Women's education must therefore be more formal, and educators have to work creatively in order to make that education realistic and relevant. This, coupled with new ways of providing woman-friendly environments for birth (in midwife-led units and birth centres) and the reinstatement of old environments (home) may herald an era in which women rediscover their power to give birth and the health service discovers the savings it can make both in the short term (fewer caesarean sections; shorter hospital stays) and long term (less maternal psychological and physical morbidity) by supporting a non-medical model of childbirth:

> *Unrestrained by fetal monitors, intravenous devices, and confinement to bed, women respond by changing positions, rocking, walking, rubbing, massaging and moaning. Women try any number of things, eventually figuring out what works best. And as women get comfortable, try to feel better, and actively 'do something', their contractions gain strength, the cervix stretches, and the baby settles into the pelvis, rotates, descends through the birth canal, and is born. Focused awareness, responding to what she is feeling, and finding a rhythm evolves as the woman experiences the pain of labor. Knowing what to do, often without thinking about it, is inner wisdom at its best. (Lothian, 1999: ix)*

> *For two hours, I continued to have contractions, which I found not too painful if I marched up the stairs at the start of each one ... By about 7.30a.m., the contractions were getting really strong and I was practically leaping up the stairs with each one. It sounds odd, and I must have taken thousands of steps that night, but it was a fantastic relief. (Woman having her first baby: personal communication, 2003)*

Teaching women how to cope physically with the pain of labour has moved on since Grantley Dick-Read's *Childbirth without Fear* was first published in 1942, and his ideas incorporated into the Natural Childbirth Trust's programme of antenatal education in 1956. The centrality of relaxation techniques to antenatal education has been challenged, and many teachers now feel that visualisation and meditation techniques may be of service only to a small minority of women. Spiby et al, (1999) express concern about continuing to teach relaxation techniques within the antenatal programme:

> *Whilst courses of preparation for labour are commonly referred to as 'relaxation classes', it is worth noting that a relatively low proportion of the sample used relaxation, given that they were members of a highly prepared and motivated group. A picture is emerging about women's views of relaxation. Women feel less confident about relaxation than the other two strategies studied (breathing and postural change) (p392).*

Relaxation cannot be taught in isolation from other coping strategies. The teaching of practical, self-help skills for labour requires a holistic approach where the woman and her birth companion are helped to understand how emotional and physical support of the woman combine with her use of posture, breathing patterns and monitoring tension in key muscle groups to assist the labour process. Teaching breathing techniques comes after the educator has helped women understand how the movement of the chest and diaphragm is affected by posture. Deep breathing and sighing out are experienced differently when the woman is standing from when she is lying on her side or leaning over a beanbag. Changing position in a hospital delivery room presents different challenges from changing position in a room in the woman's own home, or in a low-tech delivery room at a birth centre. Women also need to understand how they can use relaxation techniques in the environment where they will be labouring and this is best achieved by delivering a class or classes in that environment (see Chapter 6). The days of the isolated relaxation class with rows of women lying in semi-recumbent positions in the parentcraft room, visualising seaside scenes, are certainly long gone.

Where traditional childbirth and parenting education programmes have been based on behaviourist learning theory which sees the learner as a blank sheet upon which the educator can write her chosen script, educators must now recognise that parents-to-be are complex learners, at different stages of their physical, emotional and spiritual growth. The experience they are about to go through is one of the richest they will ever have, and antenatal education aims to maximise the potential of each individual for growing through that experience in every aspect of their being. This is the agenda for today's' responsible childbirth educator.

REFERENCES

Barlow J, Coren E, Stewart-Brown S 2002 Meta-analysis of the effectiveness of parenting programmes in improving maternal psychosocial health. British Journal of General Practice March:223-233

Brockington I 1996 Motherhood and mental health. Oxford University Press, Oxford

Bryan A A 2000 Enhancing parent – child interaction with a prenatal couple intervention. Maternal Child Nursing 25(3):139-144

Campion M J 1997 Birthcoaching: women with learning disabilities. Disability, Pregnancy and Parenthood International 17(January):13-14

Caplan H L, Coghill S R, Alexandra H 1989 Maternal postnatal depression and the emotional development of the child. British Journal of Psychiatry 154:818-822

Dick-Read G 1954 Childbirth without fear: the principles and practice of natural childbirth. Heinemann Medical Books, London

Freire P 1972 Pedagogy of the oppressed (translated by Myra Bergman Ramos). Herder and Herder, New York

Hancock A 1994 How effective is antenatal education? Modern Midwife 4(5):13

Haskins Westmoreland M, Zwelling E 2000 Developing a family-centered, hospital-based perinatal education program. The Journal of Perinatal Education 9(4):28-39

Jansen P, Blizzard S 1999 Childbirth education: does it meet women's needs? Open Line: Australian College of Midwives (Victoria Branch) 7(4):1, 10-11

Knowles M 1984 Introduction to andragogy in action. Jossey-Bass, London

Lothian J A 1999 Really teaching Lamaze: the power of pain. The Journal of Perinatal Education 8(2):viii-x

Lothian J A 2001 Really teaching Lamaze: evidence-based practice. The Journal of Perinatal Education 10(1):viii-xi

Maushart S 1997 The mask of motherhood. Vintage, Australia

Muller-Staffelstein T 1996 Preparation for childbirth – preparation for life: a challenge for primary prevention. International Journal of Prenatal and Perinatal Psychology and Medicine 8(Suppl):73-79

Rolls C, Cutts D 2001 Pregnancy-to-parenting education: creating a new approach. Birth Issues 10(2):53-59

Ross M K 2001 Promoting the transition to first-time parenthood. British Journal of Midwifery(suppl) 9(9):562-566

Sagady M 2001 The preventable caesarean section: new distinctions and new possibilities. International Journal of Childbirth Education 15(3):29-31

Schmied V, Myors K, Wills J et al 2002 Preparing expectant couples for new-parent experiences: a comparison of two models of antenatal education. The Journal of Perinatal Education 11(3):20-27

Schneider Z 2001 Antenatal education classes in Victoria: what the women said. Australian College of Midwives Incorporated 14(3):14-21

Shaull R 1972 Preface In: Freite P Pedagogy of the oppressed. Herder and Herder, New York

Sims-Jones N, Graham S, Crowe K et al 1999 Prenatal class evaluation. International Journal of Childbirth Education 13(3):29-32

Smith N 1999 Men in antenatal classes. Teaching the whole birth thing. The Practising Midwife 2(1):23-26

Spiby H, Henderson B, Slade P at al 1999 Strategies for coping with labour: does antenatal education translate into practice? Journal of Advanced Nursing 29(2):388-394

Underdown A 1998 Investigating techniques used in parenting classes. Health Visitor 71:65-66

Wilkerson N N 2000 Perspectives on learning for childbirth educators. The Journal of Perinatal Education 9(3):11-21

Index

Page numbers in bold refer to illustrations and tables

G

gender role shift 51
generalisation, using to develop curriculum 29
Gesellschaft für Geburtsvorbereitung 4–5
grape-peeling analogy in learning 34–6
group working 28
  on birth ideas workshops 94
  feedback 29
  group-building activities 24
  interaction 81
  as peer support 111

H

health care decisions by men following birth 63
health professionals
  attitude to teenage pregnancies 118
  as facilitators 129
  involved in classes 113
  see also specific people, e.g. midwives
health promotion campaigns 129
health visitors 54–5, 78
home births see childbirth, home
hope/fear exercises 24
hospital births see childbirth, hospital
hospital methods, childbirth education and 12
human cooperative behaviour 22
human psychology, study of 21–2
Hutcheson, Francis 22

I

icebreaker exercises in class 24
Indian women, perinatal mortality in **104**
infant feeding 70–1
infants
  benefit from father's involvement 59–60
  Brazleton method of assessment 64
  care, empathy-based 53
  development, information on 55
  fathers' fears of handling 60–1
informed choice 135
instruction, purpose 35
interventions see labour, interventions

K

Kolb Learning Cycle 26, 27, 30
Kolb Learning Inventory 26–30

L

labour
  alternative positions for birthing 99, 138
  coping 45–6
  curriculum 10
  father-friendly 59
  fetal positioning and 97
  innate ability of women 45
  interventions
    childbirth education and 7, 8, 12
    considered as 'normal' 39
    men questioning 58–9
    questions about 95
    rising tide 48
    teaching about 87
    see also pain relief during birth
  men's needs for guidance on 9
  partner support during 57
  questions about 96–7
  roles of men during 57
  vision of 'correct' 89
  see also delivery suite tours
Lamaze method of teaching 3–4
  importance of emotional and physical support during birth 5–6
learners see adult learners
learning see adult learning

M

marital status and labour interventions 7
Maslow, Abraham 21–2
Maslow's hierarchy of needs 21–3, 22
massage skills by fathers 58
meditation methods 137
men
  Albany Practice childbirth education groups 110
  building confidence and competence 65–6
  diffidence 61
  empowerment 58–9
  expectations from childbirth education 9, 53
  fears of handling infants 60–1
  involvement at home 59–62
  involvement in hospital 60

key concerns over pregnancy 55
  male midwives for 119
  needs 134–5
  practising infant care 61
  roles
    as breadwinners 62
    deficit perspective 65
    dissatisfaction of own and partner's 63
    as fathers 51–2, 62–4
    during labour 57, 58
    as 'playmates' 63–4
    as protectors/disciplinarians 64
  supporting 52–3
    during labour 59
    during pregnancy 55
  worries on relationships after childbirth 10
mental health of mother links to child health 134
MIDIRS Informed Choice Leaflets 37
The Midwife's Rules and Code of Practice 77
midwives
  advice 44
  anti-change 98–9
  care offered to women 5–6
  constraints on practice 72–3
  education 78
    for birth ideas workshops 92, 99
    course development 80–1
  empowerment 69–83, 86
  facilitating birth ideas workshops 92
  history of specialism 44
  involvement in Sampad 107–9
  male 119
  oppressed 72–3
  pressures to conform 74
  recognising importance of fathers 52
  role 19, 76, 77
    as facilitators 110, 118
    as specialists 77
  skills 77
  socialisation of teaching and learning methods 24
  for South Asian women 104
  style of teaching 69
  vs policy makers 86
  women's expectation and experiences 6, 6–7, 46
  see also health professionals
The Midwives Book 44

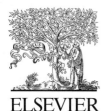

ELSEVIER

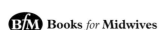 **Books** *for* **Midwives**

 CHURCHILL LIVINGSTONE   **Mosby**   THE PRACTISING MIDWIFE 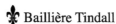 ✤ Baillière Tindall

MIDWIFERY PUBLISHERS OF CHOICE FOR GENERATIONS

For many years and through several identities we have catered for professional needs in midwifery education and practice. Leading publishers of major textbooks such as *Myles Textbook for Midwives* and *Mayes' Midwifery: a Textbook for Midwives*, our expertise spreads across both books and journals to offer a comprehensive resource for midwives at all stages of their careers.

Find out how we can provide you with the right book at the right time by exploring our website, **www.elsevierhealth.com/midwifery** or requesting a midwifery catalogue from Health Professions Marketing, Elsevier, 32 Jamestown Road, Camden, London, NW1 7BY, UK Tel: 020 7424 4200; Fax: 020 7424 4420.

We are always keen to expand our midwifery list so if you have an idea for a new book please contact Mary Seager, Senior Commissioning Editor at Elsevier, The Boulevard, Langford Lane, Kidlington, Oxford, OX5 1GB, UK (m.seager@elsevier.com).

 Have you joined yet?
Sign up for e-Alert to get the latest news and information.

Register for eAlert at www.elsevierhealth.com/eAlert Information direct to your Inbox

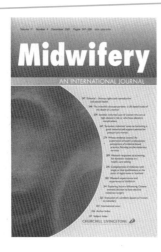

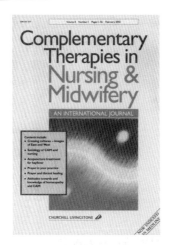

12901

Children and Adolescents With Mental Health Problems

The Library
Education Centre, Royal Surrey County Hospital
Egerton Road, Guildford, Surrey GU2 7XX
Tel: 01483 464137

Class no: WS 350   Computer no: 9804018